T0319043

When Health Care Employees Strike

When Health Care Employees Strike

A Guide for Planning
and Action

Second Edition

Kenneth F. Kruger

Norman Metzger

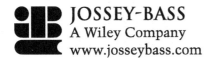

JOSSEY-BASS
A Wiley Company
www.josseybass.com

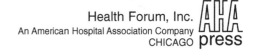

Health Forum, Inc.
An American Hospital Association Company
CHICAGO press

Published by

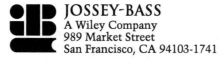

JOSSEY-BASS
A Wiley Company
989 Market Street
San Francisco, CA 94103-1741

www.josseybass.com

Jossey-Bass books and products are available through most bookstores. To contact Jossey-Bass directly, call (888) 378-2537, fax to (800) 605-2665, or visit our website at www.josseybass.com.

Substantial discounts on bulk quantities of Jossey-Bass books are available to corporations, professional associations, and other organizations. For details and discount information, contact the special sales department at Jossey-Bass.

We at Jossey-Bass strive to use the most environmentally sensitive paper stocks available to us. Our publications are printed on acid-free recycled stock whenever possible, and our paper always meets or exceeds minimum GPO and EPA requirements.

Library of Congress Cataloging-in-Publication Data

Kruger, Kenneth F.
    When health care employees strike : a guide for planning and action / Kenneth F. Kruger,
    Norman Metzger.— 2nd ed.
        p. ; cm. — (The Jossey-Bass health series)
    Metzger's name appears first on the earlier edition.
    Includes bibliographical references and index.
    ISBN 0-7879-6100-0 (alk. paper)
        1. Strikes and lockouts—Hospitals—Law and legislation—United States. 2. Collective labor
    agreements—Hospitals—United States. I. Metzger, Norman, 1924- II. Title. III. Series.
    KF3452.H6 M47 2002
    344.73'01892'61—dc21   2001007678

SECOND EDITION

PB Printing   10 9 8 7 6 5 4 3 2 1

Contents

Acknowledgments

SINCE THE PUBLICATION of the first edition of this book, the authors have experienced a forty-seven-day strike, numerous strikes of shorter duration, and more frequent use of the strike by nurses' unions. These experiences were the impetus for this second edition.

This book would not have been possible without the contributions of Joseph M. Ferentino, who coauthored the first edition. The authors also wish to acknowledge the work of Claudia McAlman and the late Irene Wehr, who worked diligently in editing and transcribing the first edition.

Special thanks to Aleida Lugo, whose assistance and dedication in helping the authors put together this second edition were invaluable.

About the Authors

KENNETH F. KRUGER serves as president of the Healthcare Human Resources Consulting Consortium, LLC, an association of respected professionals in human resource management and labor relations and Executive Healthsearch. He is a senior executive with a consistent record of accomplishment in the areas of human resources and labor relations. Kruger has a reputation as a builder, visionary, strategic planner, and problem solver with proven expertise and success in negotiating, delivering quality service, and developing and implementing effective policies and programs designed to meet organizational objectives in a changing environment.

As vice president for human resources and labor relations at the Mount Sinai Medical Center in New York City, he acted as chief spokesperson in the negotiation of numerous collective bargaining agreements. Some of his key accomplishments are the establishment of successful incentive pay programs in a unionized environment, design and implementation of a flexible benefits program that was well received by the employees and significantly reduced costs, and the establishment of an award-winning wellness program that resulted in a revenue-producing corporate product. He is highly regarded in his field, holding trusteeships in a number of union benefit funds and leadership positions in a wide range of professional associations, including past president of the American Society of Healthcare Human Resources Administration (ASHHRA). Kruger holds a master's degree in industrial and labor relations from the New York Institute of Technology and an M.B.A. degree in health services administration from Wagner College in New York.

Kruger has presented at various labor relations and human resource seminars nationwide and has written extensively in the field of human resources and labor relations. He can be contacted at http://www.healthcare hrconsulting.com or at (212) 521-4167.

NORMAN METZGER is Edmond A. Guggenheim Professor Emeritus of Health Care Management at the Mount Sinai School of Medicine. He was for many years vice president for human resources and vice president for labor relations at the Mount Sinai Medical Center in New York City. He currently serves as president of the Health Care Division of Adams, Nash, Haskell & Sheridan, Inc., a management advisory group, and as senior consultant for Martin H. Meisel Associates, an executive search company. He is a past president of the League of Voluntary Hospitals and Homes of New York and of the American Society for Healthcare Human Resources Administration (ASHHRA).

Metzger is the author, coauthor, or editor of fifteen books and has written over one hundred articles on labor relations, personnel administration, and social behavior. In 1987, he became a six-time recipient of the Annual Award for Literature given by ASHHRA in recognition for his outstanding contribution to the hospital personnel administration literature.

Metzger conducts management seminars and workshops on such subjects as empowerment, communication, transformational leadership, labor relations, interviewing skills, and motivational skills. He is a founder and was adjunct professor in the graduate program in health care administration jointly sponsored by the Mount Sinai School of Medicine and Baruch College. He has been a visiting professor at more than twenty universities.

Introduction

The strike is among the most highly publicized and the least studied social phenomena of our time.... [It] is the mechanism which produces that increment of pressure necessary to force agreement where differences are persistent and do not yield to persuasion or argument around the bargaining table.... The [alternative] to such a system might result in the demise of the collective bargaining system as we know it: some form of coercion exercised by a supreme authority, whether a government board, an industrial relations court, compulsory arbitration, or some other of the many proposals which have been advanced from time to time, would supplant the voluntarism implicit in the American collective bargaining experience. Thus, the strike, or threat of strike, is the ultimate device whereby the competing interests of antagonistic parties are expediently resolved, leading to [modi operandi that permit] both sides to accommodate their differences and live with one another.[1]

A PRIME CONCERN of health administrators in whose institutions unions begin organizational drives is the possibility of strikes. Strikes and strike threats are indeed essential parts of the total industrial collective bargaining process. Many administrators believe that recognizing a union is a direct invitation to strikes. The statistics do not confirm this theory. Nevertheless, the law does not compel parties to agree to the terms of a labor contract; rather, it only mandates that they bargain "in good faith." Unions do strike to support their positions, and management will "take a strike" in an effort to resist union demands.

In any industry, strikes put economic pressure on both parties: the workers lose wages, and the employers lose revenues. The key to a successful strike from a union's viewpoint is to inflict inordinate discomfort, expense, and pressure on the employer so as to effect a compromise or move toward the union's position. Hospital and nursing home strikes differ from those in other industries in that the resulting discomfort—and "discomfort" may be an understatement—is thrust on patients, not employers. Certainly, hospital strikes also inconvenience the public, but the greatest threat is to public health and safety. The real losers in such strikes are the patients, their families, and prospective patients (the public). The patients will be underserved: they may be moved from a struck hospital or nursing home; they may be discharged earlier than they should be. Their families will be subjected to anxiety over the limited care available and may well be forced to administer home care. Prospective patients will be troubled by the limited beds available; surgeries will be delayed, and outpatient care may be discontinued.[2]

A strike at a health care facility is the most severe form of labor-management dispute. Strikes usually produce mass picketing and sometimes violence. Such activities disrupt patient care services and result in lost revenue and bad publicity.[3]

The authors, who have been exposed over many years to strikes, walkouts, withdrawals of service, and violence on the picket line and in employee protests, have structured this book to present an overall view of strikes in the health care industry. Part One is divided into five chapters. Chapter One contains a review of the National Labor Relations Act, with a specific discourse on health care strike notice periods and remedies. The role of the Federal Mediation and Conciliation Service and boards of inquiry is discussed in relation to strike deterrence. Chapter Two defines types of strikes, from economic to unfair labor practice strikes, from sympathy strikes to violation of no-strike clauses. Chapter Three examines the strike itself, with specific emphasis on union actions and management actions. Chapter Four develops the critical difference between a strike of nurses and a strike of nonnursing personnel. Chapter Five looks at the future and makes proposals for change. Part Two of the book presents a sort of strike manual that is applicable, with appropriate adaptation, to most health care facilities.

No threat to the viability of health care services in the community is more serious than a strike of health care workers, and in many ways health care facilities are more vulnerable to strikes than manufacturing facilities. Unlike non-health-related facilities, which can stock inventory, hospitals and nursing homes cannot maintain a store of patient care. Therefore, health care facilities should plan for the worst and hope for the best.

More and more people are questioning the propriety of health care facility strikes. Patients' lives often hang in the balance. The authors believe that present remedies for impasse resolution are ineffective. One of the areas they explore in this book is the viability of an approach to health care collective bargaining that minimizes the possibility of strikes while not undercutting the collective bargaining process itself.

Notes

1. Bernard Karsh, *Diary of a Strike* (Urbana: University of Illinois Press, 1958), passim.

2. Norman Metzger and Dennis D. Pointer, *Labor Management Relations in the Health Services Industry: Theory and Practice* (Washington, D.C.: Science and Health Publications, 1972), pp. 220–221.

3. Paul Monroe Heylman, "Developing a Strike Contingency Plan," in Ira Michael Shepard and A. Edward Doudera (eds.), *Health Care Labor Law* (Washington, D.C.: AUPHA Press, 1981), p. 137.

Part One

Health Care Strikes

Legal and Moral Implications

Chapter 1

The Impact of Labor Legislation on the Health Care Industry

ON JULY 26, 1974, in his last official act as president of the United States, Richard M. Nixon signed Public Law 93-360. From that moment on, labor relations in the health care industry have been subject to a complex body of statutory, administrative, and case law. All nongovernmental health care facilities (hospitals, clinics, health maintenance organizations, nursing homes, and homes for the aged) are now covered by the federal labor law, the National Labor Relations Act (NLRA).

In 1974, health care facility administrators, who had little experience with or exposure to the NLRA prior to enactment of the law, were required for the first time to operate under its complex provisions. Labor law was a topic that most administrators had had little acquaintance with during their formal training, and specialized coursework had not prepared them to deal effectively with labor law.[1] Unfortunately, not much has changed since then. Most educational programs in health care administration deal sparingly, if at all, with labor law.

To understand the subject of strikes in health care institutions, it is essential to be familiar with the provisions of the NLRA. The major provisions of P.L. 93-360, which extended coverage of the NLRA to the health care industry, were directed toward the special nature of that industry.

Impact of P.L. 93-360 on Health Facilities

Coverage

The NLRA covers any privately operated health care institution, defined as "any hospital, convalescent hospital, health maintenance organization, health clinic, nursing home, extended care facility or other institutions devoted to the care of the sick, infirm or aged person." A hospital is covered if it has a total annual business volume of $250,000 or more; the minimum for a nursing home is $100,000. The $100,000 minimum also applies to visiting nurse associations and related associations. For all other types of private health care institutions, the minimum is $250,000. Section 2 of the act still excludes public hospitals.

Contract Notice

A party to a health care facility collective bargaining agreement wishing to modify or terminate the existing agreement must serve written notice prior to modification or termination. That notice must be served ninety days before the contract expires. The Federal Mediation and Conciliation Service (FMCS) must be notified at least sixty days prior to contract modification or termination. When a health care facility negotiates for the first time with a union for a particular bargaining unit, the FMCS must receive thirty days' notice. Figures 1.1 and 1.2 depict charts developed by the FMCS to reflect the notice requirements for health care institutions for initial contract negotiations and contract renewal negotiations, respectively.

Mediation

A special provision for the health care industry requires mandatory mediation between the parties by the FMCS. The FMCS is an independent agency of the federal government established to promote labor-management peace. A stated policy of the FMCS is to attempt to prevent or minimize work stop-

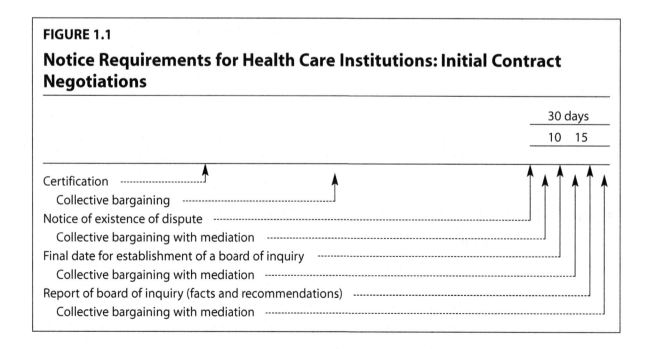

FIGURE 1.1

Notice Requirements for Health Care Institutions: Initial Contract Negotiations

30 days

10   15

Certification

Collective bargaining

Notice of existence of dispute

Collective bargaining with mediation

Final date for establishment of a board of inquiry

Collective bargaining with mediation

Report of board of inquiry (facts and recommendations)

Collective bargaining with mediation

pages in the health care industry through the use of mediation and fact-finding boards of inquiry.

After receipt of the sixty-day notice of either party, the FMCS has thirty days to decide whether to appoint a board of inquiry. Under Title 2, Conciliation of Labor Disputes in Industries Affecting Commerce, National Emergencies, a provision covering labor disputes in the health care industry has been added:

> Section 213 (a). If, in the opinion of the Director of the Federal Mediation and Conciliation Service a threatened or actual strike or lockout affecting a health care institution will, if permitted to occur or to continue, substantially interrupt the delivery of health care in the locality concerned, the Director may further assist in the resolution of the impasse by establishing within thirty days after the notice to the Federal Mediation and Conciliation Service . . . an impartial Board of Inquiry to investigate the issues involved in a dispute and to make a written report thereon to the parties within fifteen (15) days after the establishment of such a Board. The written report shall contain the findings of fact, together with the Board's recommendation for settling the dispute, with the objective of achieving a prompt, peaceful and just settlement of the dispute.

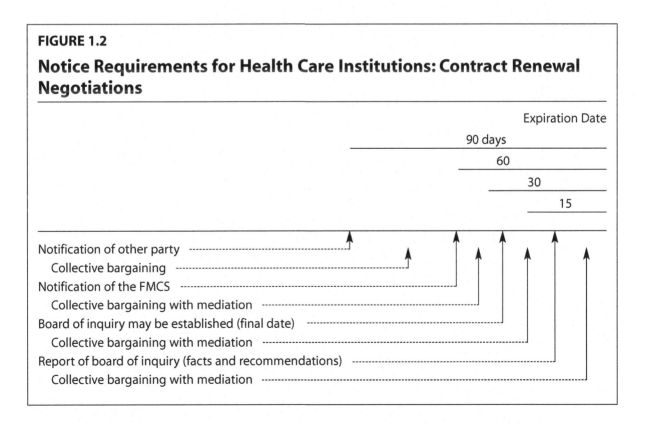

FIGURE 1.2

Notice Requirements for Health Care Institutions: Contract Renewal Negotiations

In addition, this new provision states that "after the establishment of a board . . . and for fifteen days after any such board has issued its report, no change in the status quo in effect prior to the expiration of the contract in the case of negotiations for a contract renewal, or in effect prior to the time of the impasse in the case of an initial bargaining negotiation, except by agreement, shall be made by the parties to the controversy."[2]

The board of inquiry (BOI) has fifteen days to investigate the issues and make a written report of its findings of fact and its recommendations for settling the dispute. The board's recommendations are not binding on the parties. For fifteen days after the issuance of a board report, a continued effort ensues to further negotiations and mediation, based on the BOI recommendations. No strike or lockout can legally take place until this thirty-day period ends. A board of inquiry can consist of one or more individuals. Members of such boards are not FMCS mediators but rather private arbitrators or other qualified neutrals who are selected from the FMCS official roster maintained in the FMCS Office of Arbitration Services.

In 1979, the FMCS published regulations in the *Federal Register*.[3] These regulations established that the FMCS would defer to the party's private fact-finding and interest arbitration procedures so long as they satisfy the responsibilities of the FMCS and are consistent with the NLRA. These private procedures must meet the following conditions:

- They must be invoked automatically at a specified time (e.g., at contract expiration).

- They must provide a fixed and determinate method for selecting the impartial fact finder or finders.

- They must provide that no strike or lockout take place and no change in conditions of employment (except by mutual agreement) be made prior to or during the fact-finding and for at least seven days after the procedure is completed.

- They must provide that the fact finders will make a written report to the parties, containing the findings of fact and recommendations for settling the dispute; a copy of this report must be forwarded to the FMCS (the agency is empowered to pay for the services of those boards of inquiry and fact finders appointed by the FMCS, but it cannot and does not pay for a fact finder appointed under the party's own agreement).

The FMCS will defer to the party's private interest arbitration procedure and will decline to appoint a board of inquiry or fact finders if both sides have agreed in writing to their interest arbitration procedure and if the procedure provides all of the following:

- No strike or lockout can occur and no changes in conditions of employment (except by mutual agreement) can be implemented during the contract negotiations covered by the interest arbitration procedure and during any subsequent interest arbitration proceedings.

- The arbitrators' award will be final and binding on both sides.

- There will be either a fixed and determinate method for selecting the impartial interest arbitrator or arbitrators, or the arbitrators will make a written award.[4]

The typical mediation attempt includes obtaining basic information necessary to make a personal evaluation of the situation. The mediator assembles such facts as the nature of the facility; number of beds and percentage occupied; a breakdown of a bargaining unit; identification of other bargaining units and other unions in that institution; prior bargaining experience, if any; special or unique services (this becomes an important identification preceding the decision to establish a board of inquiry); and other health care institutions in the locality, including the number of beds and special services provided by such facilities. The mediator comments on the status of negotiations and makes a recommendation regarding the appointment of a board. The FMCS regional director reviews the mediator's report and makes a recommendation to the FMCS director and to the health care coordinator in the agency's national office as to whether to appoint a board of inquiry.[5]

In many cases, contract talks are slow and may not have moved to a point where the appointment of a board would be helpful. Fully aware of this possibility, the FMCS provides for the use of a joint stipulation agreement between the parties. By this agreement, the parties authorize the FMCS director to appoint a fact finder at a later date, possibly when a union serves a ten-day strike notice. Such a fact finder normally operates under the same time limits and procedures as a board of inquiry does, unless the parties and the FMCS agree to others.

The legislative history contained in the committee report accompanying the health care amendments clearly indicated the intent of Congress in enacting special emergency dispute provisions for the health care industry:

> The Conferees intend that the appointment of a board of inquiry
> shall not operate to interrupt mediation by the FMCS, which is made
> mandatory under other provisions of this legislation, and that the
> service will pursue these parallel procedures to bring a fair, prompt,
> and just settlement of any dispute. The Conferees further intend

that the board of inquiry, in formulating its recommendations for settlement of a dispute, shall take into account all those factors normally considered by similar tribunals in formulating recommendations for the settlement of labor disputes. The committee, in adding special mediation and conciliation procedures, including the board of inquiry, for the health care industry, recognizes the need for continuity of health services during labor-management disputes and that the labor organizations representing health care workers have publicly pledged their best efforts to persuade their affiliates voluntarily to avoid work stoppages through acceptance of arbitration in the event of an impasse in negotiations. Under these new procedures, it is anticipated that, in the event of such an impasse, the findings of fact and recommendations of the board of inquiry would provide the framework of the arbitrator's decision.[6]

In its published documents, the FMCS describes the preparation for board investigations and fact-finding and the mediator's role during a board of inquiry's tenure:

Fact-finding proceedings, formal or informal, are generally conducted in a manner similar to arbitration hearings. The short time span involved in these matters makes it imperative that the parties come to the hearing fully prepared to provide the BOI with all the information it needs to understand the issues and formulate its recommendations.

Such information includes: (1) written proposals and counter proposals; (2) written stipulations on all matters agreed on during direct negotiations and mediated negotiations; (3) copies of proposed contract language and copies of previous contracts between the parties; (4) copies of arbitration decisions if related to the current dispute issues; (5) all pertinent economic data, such as changes in cost of living, comparison of wages, hours and conditions of employment in the industry and in comparable areas, and such other information as is normally taken into consideration in the determination of wages, hours and conditions of employment through voluntary collective bargaining, arbitration, or otherwise between the parties or in the industry; and (6) other information the BOI determines necessary.

The parties should also insure that all required witnesses are readily available should the BOI determine to take testimony. In preparing for the proceedings, both parties may seek technical assistance from the assigned mediator.

> Depending on the circumstances of the particular dispute, the mediator may continue with his assistance concurrent with the BOI period or mediation may be suspended during this period.
>
> In many instances, the mediator may attend board of inquiry proceedings as an observer; however, he will not participate in the proceedings in any official capacity. It is FMCS policy to maintain the neutrality of the mediator, especially as he may be required to continue mediation efforts after the BOI ceases to function.
>
> If the parties do not accept the Board's recommendations, the mediator will normally use the time until the expiration of the contract to reinitiate mediation efforts.[7]

Although used frequently by the FMCS in the 1970s, board of inquiry and fact-finding boards are rarely invoked anymore.

Strike Notice

A new section added to the NLRA prohibits a labor organization from striking or picketing a health care facility without at least ten days' notice. Congress's intent when adding section 8(g) was to provide the health care institution with advance notice so as to ensure the continuity of patient care or, at the very least, lessen the impact of the intended work stoppage on such continuity. The act further states that any employees who engage in a strike within any notice period specified in the act or who engage in any strike within the appropriate period specified in section 8(g) will lose their status as employees of the employer engaged in the particular labor dispute. Interpretation in several National Labor Relations Board (NLRB) decisions relating to activities triggering section 8(g) notice has been quite strict. The board looks to the legislative history of the amendments when attempting to interpret where picketing that does not result in a work stoppage is proscribed by the section.[8] It cited the statement made by Senator Taft during the debates on the law that "hospitals are not factories. . . . Hospitals are for human beings, and actions pursuant to this legislation must take this into account." It further noted that the committee report on the 1974 amendment stated that picketing of a health care institution would in itself constitute an unusual circumstance, justifying the application of a period of less than thirty days, whereas such "unusual circumstances" in the industrial sector normally consist of violation or intimidation. The board held that Congress intended to cover such picketing regardless of its actual impact.[9]

The section 8(g) notice requirement was intended as one of the critical compromises of the normal industrial policy of broadly permitting strikes— a compromise for the health care industry, which recognized that such notice period was in the best interest of the patients of such facilities and the public at large. The NLRB has consistently protected the hospital's and, of course, the patient's rights to such notice.[10]

The NLRB has construed section 8(g) strictly and literally, without looking to the impact of the activity involved, and it has found that picketing that does not result in work stoppage requires such notice.[11] It has also found that notice must be given by unions engaged in sympathy picketing or strike.[12] The board has ruled that notice is not required where unorganized employees are involved. It stated that the notice requirements of section 8(g) are for unions, not employees, and that the failure of employees to give such notice leaves their activity protected.[13] The board also does not require a section 8(g) notice for a threat to strike.[14] The impact of a union's conduct does not limit the board's finding violations of section 8(g).[15] It does not matter whether the object of the picketing is representational or appropriate for resolution by the FMCS. Such activity will be construed as requiring a section 8(g) notice.[16] Although the board initially found that picketing that solely involved construction work at a hospital was covered by the notice provisions,[17] the courts subsequently found that the requirements were meant to apply only to health care employees, not to employees already covered by the act.[18]

In *Montefiore Hospital and Medical Center* v. *NLRB*,[19] the U.S. Court of Appeals for the Second Circuit concurred with the holdings of other circuits that the statutory requirements of section 8(g) for a labor organization to provide a hospital with ten days' notice of its intention to engage in a strike, picketing, or other concerted refusal to work does not apply to actions by individual employees. In this decision, the court nevertheless made it clear that not every work stoppage without proper notice is permissible under the act. If such action endangers the care of patients, the court stated that it would rule that such action is unprotected and that the employees may be disciplined. The court gave the example of an emergency room personnel walkout, leaving people in need of immediate treatment. The court made it clear that each case should be viewed on its own facts and decided as to whether the employees' action places patient care in jeopardy. In this case, the court also clarified what a hospital may do to protect itself against precipitous actions by employees. The court stated that when a hospital is given notice of a union's intention to strike, "the hospital would be well advised to inquire of the rest of its employees whether they plan to stay out in sympathy. An employee who strikes after promising to show up may well forfeit protection under the Act." Within the context of this court's directive, it would be permissible for a hospital to inquire whether the employee intends to work in the event of a strike or picket, but it would be unlawful to attach any condition of employment to the employee's response. The court added that it might be lawful for a hospital to enter into "a contractual agreement not to strike without notice" with employees. Apparently, however, this ruling would be limited to physicians, registered nurses, and other professionals who serve in vital patient care capacities.

The Ally Doctrine

The Ally Doctrine is a legal doctrine developed from NLRB case law. It defines the rights of third parties who provide assistance to an employer involved in a labor dispute.[20] The doctrine affects a secondary employer who during the course of a labor dispute performs work that would have been performed by striking employees of the primary employer. In doing such work, the secondary employer loses neutral status and is therefore subject to the labor organization involved in the dispute, thus extending its economic activity to the secondary employer. As the reports of both houses of Congress in the deliberations regarding the amendments state, "It is the sense of the committee that where such secondary institutions accept the patients of a primary employer, or otherwise provide life-sustaining services to the primary employer, by providing the primary employer with an employee or employees who possess critical skills such as EKG Technician, such conduct shall not be sufficient to cause the secondary employer to lose its neutral status."[21] In effect, Congress intended to permit a neutral hospital to accept the patients of a primary employer and thereby not lose its status as a neutral.

Such a neutral hospital would, however, lose its status if it supplied *noncritical* personnel to a hospital experiencing a strike or if it not only accepted patients from such a hospital but also greatly expanded its noncritical staff in the process. Gradually, the Board's exception to the Ally Doctrine for the health care industry has become dependent on the *urgency* of the medical needs of the patients who were transferred from the primary hospital to the neutral hospital.

The 1974 Health Care Amendments to the NLRA

The 1947 Taft-Hartley Act excluded from the definition of "employer" private not-for-profit hospitals and health care institutions. The NLRB asserted jurisdiction over proprietary hospitals and nursing homes, but it was not until the 1974 amendments that Congress, through P.L. 93-360, brought the private not-for-profit health industry within the jurisdiction of federal labor law. The 1974 amendments enacted the following changes:

- The exemption contained in section 2(2) of the federal statute that excluded not-for-profit hospitals from the definition of "employer" was removed.

- A new section 2(14) was added to define the term *health care institution*. It included any "hospital, convalescent hospital, health maintenance organization, health clinic, nursing home, extended care facility or other institutions devoted to the care of sick, infirm or aged persons." This definition is essential in the determination of which employees would thereafter fall under the special health care provisions and within the scope of the act.

- A new series of special notices applicable to the health care industry and unions representing employees in that industry was enacted. The section 8(d) notice period for notices of disputes, which by law must be given by one party to the other, was extended from the normal sixty days prior to contract expiration to ninety days, and notices filed with the FMCS from the normal thirty days to sixty days. In the case of initial contract disputes, notice must be given thirty days prior to any strike notice.

- A new subsection 8(g) was added to the act. It requires that a union representing employees in a health care institution give ten days' written notice to the employer and to the FMCS of its intent to engage in a strike, picketing, or other concerted refusal to work.

- Broader sanctions under section 8(d) of the act provided that employees represented by labor organizations who do not comply with the requirements of the ninety- and sixty-day dispute notices or with section 8(g), Strike Notices, would lose their protected status under the act.

- Mandatory mediation of disputes in the health care industry were provided under section 8(d). The FMCS must mediate health care disputes, and the parties involved in such disputes are compelled to participate in that mediation process. A party's failure to participate in such mediation constitutes an unfair labor practice.

- Section 213, the second special dispute resolution provision, provided that in disputes that threaten substantial interruptions of delivery of health care in a community, the director of the FMCS may appoint a special board of inquiry to investigate the issues in the dispute and to issue publicly a written report on the dispute.

- A new section 19 provided for an alternate to the payment of union dues by persons with religious convictions against making such payments. It allows contribution to designated 501(c)(3) charities in lieu of dues.

Guidelines for Serving Section 8(g) Notices

In an interpretation by the Office of the General Counsel of the NLRB, the following guidelines have been established regarding section 8(g) notices:

- The notice should be served on someone designated to receive such notice or through whom the institution will actually be notified.

- The notice should be personally delivered or sent by mail or telegram.

- The ten-day period begins upon receipt by the employer and the FMCS of the notice.

- The notice should specify the dates and times of the strike and picketing, if both are being considered.

- The notice should indicate which units will be involved in the planned action.

As with section 8(d) notices, workers engaged in a work stoppage in violation of the ten-day strike notice lose their status as employees. The Board will probably interpret violations of the section 8(g) notice requirement as a separate and distinct unfair labor practice.

In considering the 1974 amendments to the NLRA, the congressional committee included the ten-day section 8(g) strike and picket notice to provide health care institutions with sufficient advance notice of a strike. The committee realized, however, that it would be unreasonable to expect a labor organization to commence job action at the precise time specified in a notice provided to the employer. On the other hand, if a labor organization failed to act within a reasonable period after the time specified in the notice, such action would not be in accordance with the intent of the provision. Therefore, the committee report of the amendments provided that "it would be unreasonable, in the committee's judgment, if a strike or picketing commenced more than 72 hours after the time specified in the notice. In addition, since the purpose of the notice was to give a health care institution advance notice of the actual commencement of a strike or picketing, if a labor organization does not strike at the time specified in the notice, at least 12 hours' notice should be given on the actual time for commencement of the action."

Thus, absent unusual circumstances, a union would violate section 8(g) if it struck a facility more than seventy-two hours after the designated notice time unless the parties agreed to a new time or the union gave a new ten-day notice. Furthermore, if the union does not start the job action at the designated time as provided in the initial ten-day notice, it is required to provide the health care facility at least twelve hours' notice prior to actual commencement of the action. The twelve-hour warning must fall entirely within the seventy-two-hour notice period.

The committee reports note that "repeatedly serving ten-day notices upon the employer is to be construed as constituting evidence of a refusal to bargain in good faith by the labor organization"—a violation of section 8(b)(3). What constitutes "repeatedly serving notice" will have to be defined and interpreted by the NLRB in individual cases. In a memorandum, the Board's general counsel provided the following guidelines to regional offices regarding the handling of intermittent strikes or picketing situations:

> 1. Where the facts and circumstances of the labor organization strike or picketing hiatus support the reasonable conclusion that the activity has not indefinitely ceased and that it is reasonable to assume that it will commence again, no new notice will be required if the activity recommences within 72 hours of the start of the hiatus; but 12 hours' notice to the institution will be required if the activity is to recommence more than 72 hours from the start of the hiatus.

> 2. Where the facts and circumstances of the hiatus support the reasonable conclusion that the activity has ceased indefinitely and that it will not be resumed in the near future, 12 hours' notice to the institution will be required if the activity is to resume within 72 hours of the start of the hiatus, but a new 10-day notice meeting all of the requirements of Section 8(g) will be required if the activity is to resume more than 72 hours from the start of the hiatus.

Exceptions to the requirements that labor organizations provide section 8(g) notices are indicated in two situations. First, if the employer has committed serious or flagrant unfair labor practices, notice would not be required before the initiation of the job action. Second, the employer is not allowed to use the ten-day notice period to "undermine the bargaining relationship that would otherwise exist." The facility would be free to receive supplies, but it would not be "free to stock up on the ordinary supplies for an unduly extended period"or to "bring in large numbers of supervisory help, nurses, staff and other personnel from other facilities for replacement purposes." The committee reports held that employer violation of the stated principles would release the union from its obligation not to engage in a job action during the section 8(g) notice period.

Notes

1. Dennis D. Pointer and Norman Metzger, *The National Labor Relations Act: A Guidebook for Health Care Facility Administrators* (New York: Spectrum, 1975), pp. 1–2.

2. Nancy Connolly Fibish, "The Board of Inquiry: A New Dimension in Private Sector Health Care Collective Bargaining," in Norman Metzger (ed.),

Handbook of Health Care Human Resources Management (Rockville, Md.: Aspen, 1981), p. 754.

3. "Rules and Regulations," *Federal Register,* 44, no. 14 (July 20, 1979), pp. 42683–42684.

4. Fibish, "The Board of Inquiry."

5. Fibish, "The Board of Inquiry."

6. R_x *for Labor Peace—FMCS: Its Role in the Health Care Industry,* Publication no. 0-303-728 (Washington, D.C.: U.S. Government Printing Office, 1979), p. 10.

7. R_x *for Labor Peace,* p. 12.

8. Donald A. Zimmerman, "Trends in National Labor Relations Board Health Care Industry Decisions," in Ira Michael Shepard and A. Edward Doudera (eds.), *Health Care Labor Law* (Washington, D.C.: AUPHA Press, 1981), pp. 13–16.

9. *District 1199, National Union of Hospital and Health Care Employees (United Hospitals of Newark),* 232 NLRB 443 (1977), enfd. No. 77-2472 (3d Cir. Aug. 11, 1978).

10. *Local Union 200, General Service Employees Union and Eden Park Management, Inc. d/b/a Eden Park Nursing Home and Health Rehabilitation Facility, Poughkeepsie, New York,* 263 NLRB 16. The NLRB, in a 3-to-2 decision, held that the union violated the notice provisions by participating in a sympathy strike; it joined a picket line set up by another union at a nursing home without first giving the required ten days' notice to the facility and the FMCS. The NLRB determined that the purpose of the union's picketing was "to lend support and assistance to, as well as generate publicity for, the Local 144 employees." It therefore determined that the union's action was a sympathy strike. The union's position was that it was not the certified collective bargaining representative of any employee at the nursing home and hence had no bargaining rights under the NLRA. It reasoned in defense of its action that it was not obligated to give notice in those circumstances. It said that its action was an "informal" showing of support for another union and that the notice requirements under section 8(g) were not intended to cover such limited and informal action. The NLRB, in its majority decision, found that "irrespective of its character, objectives, or the type of economic pressure it generates, any strike, work stoppage, or picketing, including sympathy picketing at a health care institution, violates Section 8(g) if the ten-day notice requirements of that Section have not been fulfilled." The board's reasoning is most important to health care facilities in this case. It flowed from the majority interpretation that the notice provisions were intended to give health care institutions sufficient time to make appropriate arrangements for continuing patient care during a labor dispute. It therefore reasoned that the necessity for complying with the notice requirement is not eliminated by the fact that the picketing labor organization does not represent the facility's

employees. To find otherwise, the board stated, would be to ignore the potential for unexpected disruption in health care service resulting from the addition of a second labor organization to the picketing activity.

11. *District 1199, National Union of Hospital and Health Care Employees (United Hospitals of Newark).*

12. *District 1199, National Union of Hospital and Health Care Employees (Retail, Wholesale and Department Store Union) (First Health Care Corporation d/b/a Parkway Pavilion Health Care),* 22 NLRB 212 (1976), enf. den. No. 76-407 (2d Cir., Nov. 23, 1976).

13. *Walker Methodist Residence,* 227 NLRB 1630 (1977); *East Chicago Rehabilitation Center, Inc.,* 252 NLRB 135 (1982) (union had no prior notice of employees' walkout); *Barry S. Solof, M.D., a Professional Corporation, d/b/a The Victoria Medical Group and the West Jefferson Medical Group,* 264 NLRB 19 (1982).

14. *Greater Pennsylvania Avenue Nursing Center, Inc.,* 227 NLRB 132 (1976).

15. *District 1199, National Union of Hospital and Health Care Employees, Retail, Wholesale and Department Store Union, AFL-CIO (South Nassau Communities Hospital),* 256 NLRB (1981).

16. *St. Joseph's Hospital Corporation,* 260 NLRB 89 (1982).

17. *United Association of Journeymen and Apprentices of the Plumbing and Pipefitting Industry of the United States and Canada, Local 630, AFL-CIO (Lein-Steenberg),* 219 NLRB 837 (1975), enf. den. 567 F.2d 1006 (D.C. Cir. 1977).

18. *Laborers' International Union of North America, AFL-CIO, Local Union No. 1057 (Mercey Hospital of Laredo) v. NLRB,* 567 F.2d 1006 (D.C. Cir. 1977); *NLRB v. International Brotherhood of Electrical Workers, Local Union No. 388 (Hoffman Company),* 548 F.2d 704 (7th Cir. 1977), cert. den. 434 U.S. 837 (1977).

19. *Montefiore Hospital and Medical Center v. NLRB,* CA 2 Nos. 79-4156 and 79-4184 (Apr. 28, 1980).

20. G. Roger King and William J. Emanuel, "Legal Developments Under the Health Care Amendments, " in Norman Metzger (ed.), *Handbook of Health Care Human Resources Management* (Rockville, Md.: Aspen, 1981), p. 580.

21. S. Rep. No. 93-766, 93d Cong. 2d sess. 5 (1974); H.R. Rep. No. 93-051, 93d Cong. 2d sess. 7 (1974).

TABLE 1.1

Work Stoppages Involving One Thousand Workers or More, 1947–1999

Year	Stoppages		Days Idle	
	Number	Workers Involved (thousands)	Number (thousands)	Percent of Estimated Working Time[a]
1947	270	1,629	25,720	N.A.
1948	245	1,435	26,127	.22
1949	262	2,537	43,420	.38
1950	424	1,698	30,390	.26
1951	415	1,462	15,070	.12
1952	470	2,746	48,820	.38
1953	437	1,623	18,130	.14
1954	265	1,075	16,630	.13
1955	363	2,055	21,180	.16
1956	287	1,370	26,840	.20
1957	279	887	10,340	.07
1958	332	1,587	17,900	.13
1959	245	1,381	60,850	.43
1960	222	896	13,260	.09
1961	195	1,031	10,140	.07
1962	211	793	11,760	.08
1963	181	512	10,020	.07
1964	246	1,183	16,220	.11
1965	268	999	15,140	.10
1966	321	1,300	16,000	.10
1967	381	2,192	31,320	.18
1968	392	1,855	35,367	.20
1969	412	1,576	29,397	.16
1970	381	2,468	52,761	.29
1971	298	2,516	35,538	.19
1972	250	975	16,764	.09
1973	317	1,400	16,260	.08
1974	424	1,796	31,809	.16
1975	235	965	17,563	.09
1976	231	1,519	23,962	.12
1977	298	1,212	21,258	.10
1978	219	1,006	23,774	.11
1979	235	1,021	20,409	.09
1980	187	795	20,844	.09
1981	145	729	16,908	.07
1982	95	656	9,061	.04
1983	81	909	17,461	.08

	Stoppages		Days Idle	
Year	**Number**	**Workers Involved (thousands)**	**Number (thousands)**	**Percent of Estimated Working Time[a]**
1984	62	376	8,499	.04
1985	54	324	7,079	.03
1986	69	533	11,861	.05
1987	46	174	4,481	.02
1988	40	118	4,381	.02
1989	51	452	16,996	.07
1990	44	185	5,926	.02
1991	40	392	4,584	.02
1992	35	364	3,989	.01
1993	35	182	3,981	.01
1994	45	322	5,020	.02
1995	31	192	5,771	.02
1996	37	273	4,889	.02
1997	29	339	4,497	.01
1998	34	387	5,115	.02
1999	17	73	1,996	.01

Notes: Stoppages and workers are counted in the year in which the stoppages began. Days of idleness include all stoppages in effect. Workers are counted more than once if they are involved in more than one stoppage during the year.   N.A. = not available.

[a]Working time is for all employees except those in private households, forestry, and fisheries.

Source: Bureau of Labor Statistics.

Chapter 2

Types of Strikes
Causes and Characteristics

ALL STRIKES are basically the same in that they are all concerted refusals of employees to continue work unless or until their employers comply with their demands.

The Taft-Hartley Act, passed in 1947 and amended in 1974, had a two-sided impact on strikes. Certain types of strikes became unlawful, while employees involved in other types of strikes were extended protection. The degree of protection depends on the type of strike. The various types include economic, unfair labor practice, sympathy, jurisdictional, recognition, and "illegal" strikes.

Economic Strikes

Economic strikes are usually conducted by the employees of a particular business who hope to compel their employer to accept their demands by withdrawing their services. Economic strikes generally occur after a breakdown in the collective bargaining process, either for the development or for the modification of a contract. The Taft-Hartley Act established specific procedures that should be followed before a party engages in a strike in these situations.

According to the 1947 act, in situations where a contract is being modified or terminated, the other party must be notified in writing sixty days prior to the modification or termination date; the Federal Mediation and Conciliation Service (FMCS) must be notified thirty days prior to this date. The 1974 amendments extended these time periods for health care institutions from sixty to ninety days for notification of the other party and from thirty to sixty days for notification of the FMCS.

The act also requires a thirty-day notice to the FMCS with regard to initial contract negotiations in health care institutions but does not require this for other industries. A ten-day notice of intent to strike must be given to health care institutions to allow them time to make arrangements for continuing patient care at their own institutions or to find other available health care providers. If a strike occurs during any of these "cooling off" periods, the strikers forfeit their status as "employees" as defined by the act and can be subject to discharge or discipline by the employer.[1] During economic strikes, employers may permanently replace strikers in order to continue business. After the strike, however, the employer must offer vacant positions, if they exist, to the strikers when they apply for reinstatement. If a striker finds equivalent employment elsewhere, the employer is no longer obligated to reinstate the striker when a vacancy occurs.[2] An employer does not have to reinstate a striker who is guilty of misconduct during a strike, even if the employee was not replaced during the strike.[3]

Unfair Labor Practice Strikes

A strike that is either caused or prolonged by the unfair labor practice of an employer is an unfair labor practice strike. Unfair labor practice strikes are afforded the highest level of protection by the National Labor Relations Board (NLRB).

Unfair labor practice strikers are entitled to unconditional reinstatement to their jobs, even if replacements must be terminated. Back pay is usually awarded from the time the strikers offer an unconditional request for reinstatement.[4]

Notification for unfair labor practice strikes is required only in the health care field. In situations involving health care institutions, unions must serve a ten-day strike notice when planning to protest an unfair labor practice, except where the unfair labor practice is flagrant or serious.[5]

In the 1961 case of Alan's Department Stores, Inc., a serious unfair labor practice was defined as "destructive of the foundation on which collective bargaining must rest."[6] In the case of District 1199-E, National Union of Hospital and Health Care Employees (CHC Corporation), the NLRB ruled that a ten-day notice was unnecessary. In this case, a five- to fifteen-minute walkout took place at a nursing home after it was learned that the administrator was hiding to avoid meeting with the employees' union representative about a grievance. The administrator had previously canceled numerous meetings on the same grievance. The nursing home subsequently filed an unfair labor practice charge against the union for failure to give a ten-day notice to strike.[7] The board determined that the nursing home had shown blatant disregard for the bargaining process, eliminating the need for a prior notice of the union's protest. The fact that no patient was harmed by the short work stoppage was also an important factor in the board's decision.[8]

Sympathy Strikes

The sympathy strike is fundamentally a strike by the workers of one employer or craft in support of the workers of another. A sympathy strike can also involve the refusal of one union to cross the picket line of another. Labor organizations that wish to engage in sympathy picketing must, however, provide a ten-day notice to health care institutions.

In 1953, the U.S. Supreme Court ruled in *NLRB* v. *Rockaway News Supply Company*[9] that an individual member's right to honor a picket line could be waived by a union through a general no-strike clause in a collective bargaining agreement. In this case, however, the bargaining history of the parties was important because the employer had rejected a union proposal that would allow its members to honor picket lines.[10]

In *Montana-Dakota Utilities* v. *NLRB*[11] and *News Union of Baltimore* v. *NLRB*,[12] the board maintained its position that a general no-strike clause prohibited sympathy strikes, based either on the bargaining history or on interpretation as such by the parties involved.[13]

The NLRB later abandoned its *News Union of Baltimore* position. In 1975, the Seventh Circuit took a different position in *Gary Hobart Water Corporation* v. *NLRB*,[14] indicating that unless there was clear and unmistakable language to the contrary, a no-strike clause does not waive an employee's right to respect picket lines. The court did, however, review the bargaining history to support its conclusion.[15]

In 1976, the Supreme Court held in *Buffalo Forge Company* v. *United Steelworkers*[16] that an injunction against a sympathy strike was prohibited by the Norris–La Guardia Act even though the collective bargaining agreement contained a no-strike pledge. If the employer went to arbitration and the arbitrator ruled that the strike was a breach of contract and ordered it to cease, then the employer could enjoin the sympathy strike.[17]

In a sympathy strike situation, therefore, a union might commit two wrongs: first, declining to arbitrate the issue of whether the sympathy strike itself is in violation of the no-strike clause of the collective bargaining agreement, and second, the sympathy strike being ruled a violation of the no-strike clause.[18]

If a sympathy strike is found to be in violation of the collective bargaining agreement, the employer is entitled to damages under section 301 of the Taft-Hartley Act.

Sympathy strikes that do not involve a picket line but rather are attempts by one or more unions to aid another in return for the future help of that union are usually unlawful. The courts have ruled that sympathy strikes, where no appreciable or observable economic interest exists, are an "unlawful infliction of damage, aimless and unjustifiable because of the absence of any direct economic advantages to the workers participating in it."[19] General strikes against all the industries of a given community or of workers in related industries have almost always been ruled illegal.

An example of a no-strike clause that prohibits sympathy strikes is found in the May 1, 1999, to April 30, 2002, collective bargaining agreement between the Mount Sinai Medical Center and Local Union no. 3, International Brotherhood of Electrical Workers:

Article XXIII

No Strike or Lockout

1. No Employee shall engage in any strike, sit-down, sit-in, slow-down, cessation or stoppage or interruption of work, boycott, or other interference with the operations of the Hospital.

2. The Union, its officers, agents, representatives and members, shall not in any way, directly or indirectly, authorize, assist, encourage, participate in or sanction any strike, sit-down, sit-in, slow-down, cessation or stoppage or interruption of work, boycott, or other interference with the operations of the Hospital, or ratify, condone or lend support to any such conduct or action.

3. In addition to any other liability, remedy or right provided by applicable law or statute, should a strike, sit-down, sit-in, slow-down, cessation or stoppage or interruption of work, boycott, or other interference with the operations of the Hospital occur, the Union, within twenty-four (24) hours of a request by the Hospital, shall:

   a) Publicly disavow such action by the Employees.

   b) Advise the Hospital in writing that such action by Employees has not been sanctioned by the Union.

   c) Notify Employees of its disapproval of such action and instruct such Employees to cease such action and return to work immediately.

> d) Post notices at Union Bulletin Boards advising that it dis-
> approves such action, and instructing Employees to return
> to work immediately.
>
> 4. This prohibition against strikes, work stoppages or work inter-
> ruptions shall include a prohibition against such activity
> which is directed in sympathy with other Employees or with
> other unions at Mount Sinai Medical Center and at other
> institutions.

Jurisdictional Strikes

A jurisdictional strike is a work stoppage resulting from a dispute between two or more unions over the assignment of work. If an employer assigns the work in dispute to a particular union, the other will strike.[20] Section 8(b)(4)c of the Taft-Hartley Act made it an unfair labor practice for a union to strike or cause concerted refusal to perform a service or to handle goods with the purpose of "forcing or requiring any employer to assign particular work to employees in a particular labor organization or in a particular trade, craft or class rather than to employees in another labor organization or in another trade, craft or class, unless such employer is failing to conform to an order or certification of the Board determining the bargaining representative for employees performing such work."

In jurisdictional disputes, if one union threatens a strike, either the employer or a competing union may file an unfair labor practice charge with the regional director of the NLRB. "The regional director will then issue a complaint and immediately seek a federal district court injunction against the strike."[21] The standard used to determine if an injunction will be issued is "whether the regional director has a reasonable cause to believe that a violation has occurred."[22]

Recognition Strikes

Strikes or work stoppages for the purpose of forcing an employer to bargain with a particular labor organization are recognition strikes. For the most part, labor organizations are prohibited under section 8(b)(7) of the National Labor Relations Act from picketing or threatening to picket an employer for recognition purposes if the employer has lawfully recognized any other labor organization under the provisions of the act, if a valid election has been conducted within the preceding twelve months, or if a representational petition has not been filed within a reasonable period, not to exceed thirty days from the commencement of such picketing.[23] When health care institutions are involved, the congressional committee reports encourage the NLRB to consider this an unusual circumstance and limit this thirty-day period allowed for recognitional picketing at health care facilities.[24]

When a valid charge has been filed with the NLRB concerning a recognition strike or picketing, the Board must seek an injunction under the act against the strike or picketing unless a valid charge of employer domination of a union has been filed.

Illegal Strikes

Several types of strikes are illegal. Determination of the illegality of a strike is usually based on the Taft-Hartley Act as amended and in other cases by the collective bargaining agreement. Here are some examples of illegal strikes:[25]

A sit-down strike where employees remain in the institutions and prevent work from going on

A strike that is violent

A wildcat strike (one that is not authorized by the union)

Strikes in defiance of existing certification

Jurisdictional strikes

Secondary strikes and boycotts

A strike to induce the violation of a valid statute

A strike to obtain a featherbedding arrangement

Strikes involving issues that are applicable to the grievance and arbitration procedure of a collective bargaining agreement can also be held to be illegal.

Strikes in Violation of No-Strike Clauses

Most collective bargaining agreements have some type of no-strike clause. For a union to agree to a no-strike clause, usually management must also agree to an arbitration clause. Exhibit 2.1 presents examples of no-strike and arbitration clauses.

The United States Arbitration Act supplies significant support for arbitration. First enacted on February 12, 1925, and amended on July 30, 1947, September 3, 1954, and July 31, 1970, the U.S. Arbitration Act makes arbitration agreements specifically enforceable with regard to contracts involving interstate or international commerce. The law, however, excludes "contracts of employment"; whether this excludes collective bargaining

EXHIBIT 2.1

Examples of No-Strike and Arbitration Clauses

NO STRIKE OR LOCK OUT

1. No Employee shall engage in any strike, sit-down, sit-in, slow-down, cessation or stoppage or interruption of work, boycott, or other interference with the operations of the Employer.
2. The Union, its officers, agents, representatives and members, shall not in any way, directly or indirectly, authorize, assist, encourage, participate in or sanction any strike, sit-down, sit-in, slow-down, cessation or stoppage or interruption of work, boycott, or other interference with the operations of the Employer, or ratify, condone or lend support to any such conduct or action.
3. In addition to any other liability, remedy or right provided by applicable law or statute, should a strike, sit-down, sit-in, slow-down, cessation or stoppage or interruption of work, boycott, or other interference with the operations of the Employer occur, the Union, within twenty-four (24) hours of a request by the Employer, shall:
   (a) Publicly disavow such action by the Employees.
   (b) Advise the Employer in writing that such action by Employees has not been called or sanctioned by the Union.
   (c) Notify Employees of its disapproval of such action and instruct such Employees to cease such action and return to work immediately.
   (d) Post notice at Union Bulletin Boards advising that it disapproves such action, and instructing Employees to return to work immediately.
4. The Employer agrees that it will not lock out Employees during the term of this Agreement.

ARBITRATION

1. A grievance, as defined in Article XXXI, which has not been resolved there under may, within thirty (30) working days after completion of Step 3 of the grievance procedure, be referred for arbitration by the Employer or the Union to an arbitrator selected in accordance with procedures of the American Arbitration Association. The arbitration shall be conducted under the Voluntary Labor Arbitration Rules then prevailing of the American Arbitration Association.
2. The fees and expenses of the American Arbitration Association and the arbitrator shall be borne equally by the parties.
3. The award of an arbitrator hereunder shall be final, conclusive and binding upon the Employer, the Union and the Employees.
4. The Arbitrator shall have jurisdiction only over disputes arising out of grievances, as defined in Section 1 of Article XXXI, and he/she shall have no power to add to, subtract from, or modify in any way any of the terms of this Agreement.
5. All grievances contesting a discharge referred to arbitration after the execution of this Agreement shall be conducted in accordance with the procedures of the American Arbitration Association under the Voluntary Labor Arbitration Rules then prevailing; the single panel of arbitrators shall be abolished.
6. All demands for arbitration filed after January 4, 1993 shall be subject to arbitration procedure set forth below in Paragraphs 7 through 12. To the extent that Paragraphs 7 through 12 are not implemented, the League and the Union will make a good faith effort to implement these provisions as quickly as possible.
7. The American Arbitration Association will produce one list of eleven (11) names of arbitrators, seven (7) of whom are members of the National Academy of Arbitrators, and all of whom have dates available to

hear cases within thirty (30) working days of selection. The parties will alternately strike names until one remains who shall be the arbitrator. The time period for selecting the arbitrator shall be seven (7) business days. The Employer and the Union shall strike the first name on an alternating basis.

8. The arbitration hearing shall be held within thirty (30) working days of appointment of the arbitrator or within thirty (30) working days of completion of the mediation procedure or 1199-League Grievance Committee procedure if either has been requested, whichever is later. Neither side shall be entitled to more than one (1) adjournment of that date, unless there is mutual consent. The adjourned date must be within thirty (30) working days of the postponed hearing date.

9. If the parties agree, the arbitrator shall hear more than one case in a day.

10. No briefs shall be submitted in disciplinary cases heard in one day. The parties agree in principle— and the arbitrators will be instructed—that briefing should be avoided or limited in all cases unless complexity of the issues demand briefing. In such situations, the parties must agree on the filing of briefs or obtain approval from the arbitrator to file briefs. Briefs, if permitted, are to be filed within two weeks of hearing.

11. Arbitrators' decisions are to be rendered within two (2) weeks. However, in disciplinary cases, awards shall be issued within forty-eight (48) hours with an opinion to follow.

12. Arbitrators are to be instructed to issue succinct decisions in all cases, attempting, wherever possible, to limit study and writing time to one-half (1/2) day.

Source: 1998–2001 Collective Bargaining Agreement between the League of Voluntary Hospitals and Homes of New York and Local 1199, National Health and Human Service Employees Union SEIU/AFL-CIO. Reprinted with permission.

agreements or pertains only to individual contracts of employment has been subject to dispute, with the courts issuing conflicting decisions.[26]

The 1957 Supreme Court decision in *Textile Workers* v. *Lincoln Mills*[27] is among the most important case law in this area. In that case, the High Court ruled that future dispute clauses in collective bargaining agreements could be enforced in federal courts under section 301 of the Taft-Hartley Act, thus establishing the jurisdiction of federal courts in labor matters. The federal courts could therefore invoke a remedy for the failure of the party to honor its agreement to arbitrate. This decision also paved the way for injunctions to be imposed in labor disputes where agreements exist to arbitrate grievance disputes.[28]

In *Charles Dowd Box Company* v. *Courtney*[29] and *Local 174, Teamsters* v. *Lucas Flour Company*,[30] the Supreme Court left open the possibility of state court jurisdiction in the enforcement of collective bargaining agreements as long as they adhered to federal law as indicated by the *Lincoln Mills* decision.[31]

An important decision that seems to conflict with the Norris–La Guardia Act of 1932, which specifically limits the power of federal courts to issue either temporary or permanent injunctions in nonviolent labor disputes, resulted from *Boys Markets, Inc.,* v. *Retail Clerks Local 770.*[32] The 1970 decision set forth three tests for a strike injunction:

1. The strike must concern a grievance the parties are contractually bound to arbitrate.

2. The employer, as well as the union, must be ordered to arbitrate.

3. Traditional equity principles must be satisfied.[33]

The first of the three principles left a basic question unanswered: What about the situation where the strike itself is potentially in violation of the collective bargaining agreement? This was precisely the issue in *Buffalo Forge Company* v. *United Steelworkers.*[34] This 1976 case involved a sympathy strike over an issue that was not arbitrable. In its decision, the court held that the possibility of the sympathy strike under the terms of the collective bargaining agreement must itself be decided by arbitration before an injunction could be appropriately issued.[35]

In *Cedar Coal Company* v. *UMW Local 1759,*[36] a case where the grievance causing the primary strike was arbitrable and a sympathy strike also took place to force the employer to give in on an arbitrable issue, the Supreme Court ruled in 1978 that an injunction may be issued against the primary strike as well as the sympathy strike.[37]

Notes

1. Howard J. Anderson (ed.), *Primer of Labor Relations,* 2nd ed. (Washington, D.C.: Bureau of National Affairs, 1975), p. 70.

2. Dennis D. Pointer and Norman Metzger, *The National Labor Relations Act: A Guidebook for Health Care Facility Administrators* (New York: Spectrum, 1975), p. 138.

3. Pointer and Metzger, *The National Labor Relations Act,* p. 138.

4. Anderson, *Primer of Labor Relations,* p. 67.

5. Kenneth C. McGuiness, *How to Take a Case Before the National Labor Relations Board,* 4th ed. (Washington, D.C.: Bureau of National Affairs, 1976), p. 345.

6. Douglas L. Leslie, *Labor Law* (St. Paul, Minn.: West, 1979), p. 97; *Arlan's Department Stores Inc.,* 133 NLRB 802 (1961).

7. *District 1199-E, National Union of Hospital and Health Care Employees (CHC Corporation),* 229 NLRB 15 (1979); G. Roger King and William J. Emmanuel, "Legal Developments Under the Health Care Amendments," in Norman Metzger (ed.), *Handbook of Health Care Human Resources Management* (Rockville, Md.: Aspen, 1981), p. 578.

8. *District 1199-E, National Union of Hospital and Health Care Employees (CHC Corporation);* King and Emanuel, "Legal Developments," p. 578.

9. *NLRB* v. *Rockaway News Supply Company,* 345 U.S. 71 (1953).

10. Walter B. Connolly Jr. and Michael J. Connolly, *Work Stoppages and Union Responsibility* (New York: Practicing Law Institute, 1977), pp. 212–214.

11. *Montana-Dakota Utilities* v. *NLRB,* 455 F.2d 1088 (8th Cir. 1972).

12. *News Union of Baltimore* v. *NLRB,* 393 F.2d 673 (D.C. Cir. 1968).

13. Connolly and Connolly, *Work Stoppages,* pp. 213–214.

14. *Gary Hobart Water Corporation* v. *NLRB,* 511 F.2d 284 (7th Cir. 1975).

15. Connolly and Connolly, *Work Stoppages,* pp. 214–215.

16. *Buffalo Forge Company* v. *United Steelworkers,* 428 U.S. 397, 96 S.Ct. 3141, 49 L.Ed.2d 1022 (1976).

17. Leslie, *Labor Law,* pp. 298–299.

18. Connolly and Connolly, *Work Stoppages,* p. 281.

19. Charles O. Gregory and Harold A. Katz, *Labor and the Law,* 3rd ed. (New York: Norton, 1979), p. 109.

20. Leslie, *Labor Law,* p. 176.

21. Leslie, *Labor Law,* p. 176.

22. Leslie, *Labor Law,* p. 177.

23. Pointer and Metzger, *The National Labor Relations Act,* p. 128.

24. Pointer and Metzger, *The National Labor Relations Act,* p. 59.

25. Pointer and Metzger, *The National Labor Relations Act,* p. 139.

26. Dennis R. Nolan, *Labor Arbitration Law and Practice* (St. Paul, Minn.: West, 1979), p. 39.

27. *Textile Workers* v. *Lincoln Mills of Alabama,* 353 U.S. 448 (1957).

28. Maurice S. Trotta, *Arbitration of Labor Management Disputes* (New York: AMACOM, 1974), p. 109.

29. *Charles Dowd Box Company* v. *Courtney,* 368 U.S. 502 (1962).

30. *Local 174, Teamsters* v. *Lucas Flour Company,* 369 U.S. 95 (1962).

31. Nolan, *Labor Arbitration Law and Practice,* p. 45.

32. *Boys Markets, Inc.,* v. *Retail Clerks Local 770,* 398 U.S. 235, 90 S.Ct. 1583, 26 L.Ed.2d 199 (1970).

33. Nolan, *Labor Arbitration Law and Practice,* pp. 56–57.

34. See note 16.

35. Nolan, *Labor Arbitration Law and Practice,* pp. 57–60.

36. *Cedar Coal Company* v. *UMW Local 1759,* 560 F.2d 1153 (4th Cir. 1977), cert. den. 434 U.S. 1047 (1978).

37. Nolan, *Labor Arbitration Law and Practice,* pp. 60–61.

Chapter 3

Strike-Related Actions

Union and Management

COLLECTIVE BARGAINING is the interaction between unions and management within the limits set forth by formal rules, accepted practices, laws, and conventions.[1] The primary purpose of collective bargaining is to regulate the relations between the management of an organization and its workers. Through this process, an attempt is made to establish and maintain mutually acceptable and beneficial rules and practices to guide their conduct in daily operations.[2] In most situations, labor and management will reach a mutually acceptable agreement. Occasionally, however, this agreement is reached only through a strike or, on rare occasions, a lockout. A strike at a health care facility is, of course, an extremely serious matter that can have devastating consequences. In his book *Mediation and the Dynamics of Collective Bargaining,* William E. Simkin outlined the following reasons for strikes:[3]

1. One (or both) of the parties is unable to or unwilling to make decisions required to reach agreement.

2. One (or both) of the parties is unable or unwilling to accept an alternative settlement procedure or a device for postponement of economic action.

3. The issues in conflict are so important to one (or both) parties that "a test of strength" is needed to change positions.

Strikes have a definite effect on the positions of the bargaining parties. They increase the likelihood that initial issues will change. An example is the 1980 strike at Ashtabula Hospital in Ohio by the Ohio Nurses Association, a strike that lasted 570 days (one of the longest nursing strikes on record). The issues on which this strike was settled were totally different from those that initially caused the strike. (Appendix A at the end of Part One provides a chronology of events in the Ashtabula strike.)

Strikes can also prevent negotiators from dealing with the issues that precipitated the strike because they are preoccupied with their respective roles during a strike.[4] Emotions sometimes replace reason during a strike, and positions harden. New issues may appear, and issues thought to be resolved may reappear.[5]

The ratio of strikes to the total number of health care cases completed by the Federal Mediation and Conciliation Service (FMCS) has remained relatively stable since 1974, ranging from 4.2 to 5.5 percent of the total health care cases.[6] A 1979 study conducted by Lucretia Dewey Tanner, Harriet Goldberg Weinstein, and Alice Lynn Ahmuty and financed by the Department of Labor found that nursing home strikes tend to last longer than hospital strikes, averaging fifty-two days, compared to eighteen days for hospitals. One union organizer postulated that nursing home strikes last longer because the public does not exert the same pressure to resolve disputes in nursing homes as it does in instances involving hospitals; therefore, nursing home strikes that were not settled in the first few days tended to have a long duration.[7] The 1994 Healthcare Strike Survey results prepared by the American Society for Healthcare Human Resources Administration (ASHHRA) Legislative and Labor Committee and Modern Management Inc. found that strikes were slightly shorter for hospitals, with the majority of strikes ending within two weeks.

Numerous studies have been conducted on the propensity of strikes with respect to the effect of unemployment rates, differential movements in wages and prices, and geographical factors. The occurrence of strikes varies inversely with the unemployment rate.[8] Therefore, high rates of unemployment have seriously affected the bargaining power of unions, and their inclination toward a strike is minimal.[9]

Inflation has also been found to have an impact on the number of strikes.[10] During times of high inflation, unions tend to make larger demands to increase the purchasing power of their members to "catch up" with the inflation rate, resulting in more strikes. Where wage increases exceed the inflation rate, historically there have been fewer strikes.[11]

With regard to geographical factors, studies have found that states in the South have less strike activity than other states.[12] This, of course, results from cultural, historical, and political factors that have hindered unionization in the South.[13] Studies have demonstrated that rural areas have a higher propensity to strike[14] due to minimal social outlets and lack of alternative employment opportunities "to mediate or neutralize work related conflicts and grievances."[15]

The cost of a strike to a hospital involves lost patient revenues, especially in the outpatient department and the inpatient medical/surgical units.[16] Strike-related expenses include additional costs associated with temporary or agency employees, overtime costs for nonstriking employees, security expenses (if additional security is needed), additional supplies and equipment expense (especially if disposables are substituted), food costs (if provided to working employees free or at reduced rates), and in some cases unemployment insurance costs. Also lost are less tangible management hours to such strike-necessitated functions as contingency operational planning and, to the extent possible, patient care. Legal costs associated with strike settlement efforts can be prohibitive. Patients may also seek substitute health care facilities and may not return to the struck facility. The cost of sabotage, both overt and covert, can also be significant, as can the costs of arbitrating strike-related discharge and discipline cases.

The cost of the strike to the union can also be considerable. Striking workers could be replaced, having an impact, albeit temporarily, on union dues. The struck facility might have to shut down completely, as in the case of Ashtabula General. Even if the union's members are reinstated, the union faces administrative and strike benefit costs in addition to member dissatisfaction with lost wages and fringes. The union must also consider the ramifications of an unsuccessful strike on future decertification and representation elections. A common management tactic (often used during organizing drives) is to publicize the union's strike record and the potential effects of strikes on employees, such as loss of pay and the relationship of a day of lost pay to the settlement necessary to make up for that loss.

Major Elements of Strikes in Progress

We shall now turn our attention to management and union conduct relative to strike actions, strike-related discipline, and the employee's option of resigning from the union in the event of a work stoppage, among other topics.

Preparing for the Strike

When facing the threat of a strike, management must develop a plan that will both provide care for the patients remaining in the hospital and protect nonstriking employees.

One of management's first decisions must be to determine whether the hospital will continue to operate and, if so, at what level. This decision will be determined to a large degree by the number and classifications of striking employees. A strike by service and maintenance employees, for instance, may not require a significant reduction in patient services. However, if the technical and clerical employees join the service and maintenance workers, service reduction will accelerate. A strike of nurses poses more immediate problems to hospital administrators than a strike of nonnurse personnel due to its obvious direct impact on patient care. A strike contingency plan, such as the plan outlined in Part Two of this book, is essential for health care facilities coping with a strike.

Damage Suits for Unlawful Strikes

In certain circumstances, employers may sue a labor organization for damages to business or property resulting from an illegal strike or boycott under section 303 of the Taft-Hartley Act, as amended. Some of the strikes considered illegal under section 8(b)(4) of the National Labor Relations Act (NLRA) are those involving "hot cargo" agreements, secondary strikes and boycotts, strikes in defiance of existing certification, jurisdictional strikes, sit-down strikes where employees remain in the institution and prevent work from being performed, violent strikes, and wildcat strikes. The NLRA has the following to say on this point:

> Sec. 303. (a) It shall be unlawful, for the purpose of this section only, in an industry actively affecting commerce, for any labor organization to engage in any activity or conduct defined as an unfair labor practice in section 8(b)(4) or 8(g) of the National Labor Relations Act, as amended.
>
> (b) Whoever shall be injured in his business or property by reason of any violation of subsection (a) may sue therefore in any district court of the United States subject to the limitations and provisions of Section 301 hereof without respect to the amount in controversy, or in any other court having jurisdiction of the parties, and shall recover the damages by him sustained and the cost of the suit.
>
> Sec. 301. (a) Suits for violation of contracts between an employer and a labor organization representing employees in an industry affecting commerce as defined in this Act, or between any such labor organizations, may be brought in any district court of the United States having jurisdiction of the parties, without respect to the amount in controversy or without regard to the citizenship of the parties.
>
> (b) Any labor organization which represents employees in an industry affecting commerce as defined in this Act and any employer whose activities affect commerce as defined in this Act shall be bound by the acts of its agents. Any such labor organization may sue or be sued as an entity and in behalf of the employees whom it represents in the courts of the United States. Any money judgment against a labor organization in a district court of the United

States shall be enforceable only against the organization as an entity and against its assets, and shall not be enforceable against any individual member or his assets.

(c) For the purposes of actions and proceedings by or against labor organizations in the district courts of the United States, district courts shall be deemed to have jurisdiction of a labor organization (1) in the district in which such organization maintains its principal offices, or (2) in any district in which its duly authorized officers or agents are engaged in representing or acting for employee members.

(d) The service of summons, subpoena or other legal process of any court in the United States upon an officer or agent of a labor organization, in his capacity as such, shall constitute service upon the labor organization.

(e) For the purposes of this section, in determining whether any person is acting as an "agent" of another person so as to make such other person responsible for his acts, the question of whether the specific acts performed were actually authorized or subsequently ratified shall not be controlling.

Thus under section 303 of the law, any person suffering business or property losses may sue for the damages caused by an unlawful boycott or strike. This includes customers, suppliers, and others doing business with the affected employer, as well as the employer itself. The courts, however, have declared that recovery may come only from labor organizations and not from individuals involved in unauthorized strikes.[17] "Persons suing for damages caused by unlawful strike or the coercive action can recover actual dollar-and-cents losses, plus court costs. However, they cannot collect additional amounts as penalties for malicious injury [or] to curb future misconduct. Nor can attorney fees incurred during NLRB proceedings relating to a union's unlawful secondary activity be recovered in a later suit for damages, the U.S. Supreme Court has ruled."[18]

A federal appeals court ruled that while it is true that only compensation damages can be collected under federal law, punitive damages may be collected where tactics were used in violation of state criminal law.[19] An arbitrator may also rule against a union for damages where it can be shown that the union violated a no-strike clause.

An example of such an award is *Fortex Manufacturing Company, Inc.*, v. *Local 1065, Amalgamated Clothing and Textile Workers of America.*[20] In this case, a picket line was established in violation of the no-strike clause of the collective bargaining agreement, to protest the discharge of an employee. The union's contention was that it did end the strike and that consequently the claim for damages should be dismissed. The arbitrator held, however, that the union should have taken more forceful action by disciplining the strikers as provided in the union's constitution and bylaws. The union was held liable for damages sustained, including reasonable attorney's fees, overhead expenses not offset by production, direct expenses, and overtime costs. The arbitrator also found the union liable for the arbitrator's fee and expenses.

Another example is *Foster Grading Company*.[21] In this case, the arbitrator awarded the company, which was working on a highway project, compensatory damages for "labor costs, rental value of equipment (its own and outside rentals), and the prorated costs of traffic protection."[22]

Union Actions During a Strike

When calling a strike, unions follow procedures generally outlined in their constitutions. The following is an example of a strike procedure, found in the Constitution of District 1199, National Union of Hospital and Health Care Employees:

> **ARTICLE XV—STRIKES**
>
> Section 1—The National Union shall be informed of any decision to call or terminate a strike.
>
> Section 2—A strike may be called by a District or a sub-division thereof only with the approval of the members involved at a meeting duly called to consider the matter. Such approval shall be voted on by secret ballot.
>
> Section 3—Any proposal to settle or terminate a strike shall require the approval of the membership involved at a meeting duly called to consider the matter and voted on by secret ballot.
>
> Section 4—All requests for benefits from the National Strike and Defense Fund shall be made in the first instance to the president of the National Union, who may appoint a standing committee of the National Executive Board to act upon such requests.

District 1199 has renamed itself the National Health and Human Services Employees Union and is now a local of the Service Employees International Union. Its constitution, adopted March 1985 and amended 1987, has deleted the language just cited and features the following statements in its stead:

> 1. Article VII Section 10 Executive Council   "The Executive Council shall have the following powers: to call strikes, subject to the approval of the members directly involved."
>
> 2. Article VII Section 12 Delegate Assemblies   "The Division Delegate Assembly shall have the power to call strike in its Division, subject to approval of the members directly involved."

The American Nurses Association (ANA) bargains collectively through its Economic and General Welfare Program. The program provides the necessary assistance and establishes the guidelines for the various state nurses' associations. Each state association is made up of a number of local bargaining units.

Local units must make their own collective bargaining decisions, including authorization to strike.[23] Strike authorization by the New York State Nurses Association (NYSNA), Council of Nurse Practitioners of the Mount Sinai Hospital, is subject to the following requirements:

1. A well-publicized meeting shall be held.
2. Voting shall be by open ballot.
3. Tellers shall be appointed by the chairperson prior to voting period.
4. A two-thirds (2/3) vote of the Council shall be required.
5. A NYSNA General Representative shall be in attendance at this meeting.

The Service Employees International Union (SEIU) represents employees working in hospitals, nursing homes, other health care facilities, and in non-health-related industries. To call a strike, a local of the SEIU has required the approval of its international president.[24]

The Retail Clerks International Union (RCIU) represents employees primarily engaged in the distribution or provision of consumer products. Food, apparel, shoe, hardware, furniture, and variety stores, as well as health care facilities, are considered potential areas for organization. RCIU strikes have had to be approved by two-thirds of the members involved in the strike and by the union's international president.[25]

Strike Funds

Most unions have established strike funds, which are allocated during a strike to cover strike benefits, legal fees, publicity, and other related expenses. Some unions assess each member a small amount each month to build the fund. The amount of the fund often determines the staying power of the workers and consequently the success or failure of the strike. At one time, District 1199 had a National Union Strike and Defense Fund, which could be used through a request to the president of the National Union, who might establish a standing committee of the national executive board to act on the request. The National Union allocated 10 percent of total dues, initiation fees, and assessments collected by its locals for the National Union Strike and Defense Fund. The executive board, consisting of the president, the executive vice president, the secretary-treasurer, the executive secretary, and the secretary and vice presidents of the National Union, could authorize collection of additional revenue to supplement the fund, if necessary.[26]

The revised constitution for the renamed 1199 National Health and Human Services Employees Union (SEIU) adopted March 1985 and amended November 1987, in Article 5, Section 9, Dues and Good Standing, states: "Five per cent (5%) of all dues collected shall be set aside by the Union for a Strike and Defense Fund. This amount can be adjusted based on the determination of the Executive Council and its best estimates of the Union's need in this matter."

The ANA has no general strike fund. Some state associations have established their own strike-assistance funds. The ANA will, however, assist state associations in need of additional strike funds by soliciting donations nationally.[27] The formation of the United American Nurses and the union's affiliation with the AFL-CIO in 2001 may ultimately result in the establishment of a strike fund as well as a change in the tactics employed in labor disputes.

Locals of the SEIU have been required to first obtain approval from the international president before drawing money from their own strike fund. The fund is fed by a per capita tax on the membership. During an authorized strike, each local, with presidential approval, may use the equivalent of its contributions to the fund and borrow an additional equal amount.[28]

The RCIU pays no strike benefits until the strike has continued for two weeks. These benefits come from the general fund.[29]

Strike Strategy

For a strike to be successful, the union must ensure adequate participation by membership employed at the struck facility, establish a base of operations near the site of the strike, and develop a theme or mechanism that will muster public support. Delegates and assigned union representatives will help union leaders encourage membership participation in the strike. They usually visit the target facility prior to the strike, gathering support of the membership. Flyers are normally distributed, outlining management's position in negotiations. During the strike itself, the union usually attempts to get as many organizers or business agents as possible to the strike site or appoints captains to distribute signs and organize picket lines in an attempt to maximize operational interruption and ineffectiveness while affording picketers high visibility to the public and the media.

The union will commonly establish a base of operations near the strike site, in vacant storefronts or trailers. The base serves as strike headquarters, where strike efforts are coordinated and, in some cases, coffee and food are distributed to the strikers. Of paramount concern to strike coordinators are the media—the pipeline to the public. Due to the unpopularity of strikes in the health care industry, the union must carefully develop a theme that will put management on the defensive while justifying its action to strike. The union may accuse management of trying to "bust the union" or indicate that the quality of care in the institution is poor and that the strike is an effort to improve that situation.

More sophisticated unions will employ a "corporate campaign" in addition to or in lieu of a strike. This involves using politicians, religious leaders, and the media to pressure management and possibly trustees into conceding to the union's position. Other tactics include direct contact with trustees, in an effort to find one or more who may be sympathetic, and direct contact with patients and physicians, usually stressing how management's position will affect patient care. Radio, television, and newspaper ads, along with sympathetic articles written in local newspapers, are also common.

Massive rallies to get media attention, along with the appearance of well-known personalities at the rallies or on the picket line, are also common tactics. Community groups may also be convinced or at least appear to join strikers on the picket line. Regulatory agencies are also often called during the strike to review patient care activities and safety concerns reported by the union or its agents, and unfair labor practices are filed throughout the strike for various reasons.

The use of the strike has also changed. The traditional strike without a predetermined duration is being replaced by a number of limited-duration strikes of one to three days, designed to disrupt operations while not placing striking employees in the kind of uncertain financial situation that would result from a strike of unknown duration. This tactic is frequently thwarted through the use of lockouts until an agreement is reached.

Discipline for Activity During the Strike

Violence on the picket line is not uncommon. One of the primary objectives of the picket line is to discourage people from entering the facility. In this effort, confrontations with patients, vendors, police, and others can be serious. Picketing employees are often disciplined at the conclusion of the strike for their actions while on the line. Union leaders often demand amnesty for their members as a condition of strike settlement. Management should be aware when considering such amnesty that amnesty may encourage similar violent action by striking employees in future strikes.

Union Disciplinary Action Against Its Members

Most union constitutions and bylaws provide for disciplinary action against members who violate enunciated rules or policies. Such action can be a simple reprimand or may take the form of a more serious censure, fine, suspension, or expulsion.

Employer Discipline of Striking Employees

Illegal strikes could result in management disciplinary action up to and including discharge against all strikers or at least those responsible for strike initiation or exacerbation.[30] In other strike situations, disciplinary action might be taken against one or more striking employees for individual acts of violence. Such acts should be identified by solid evidence.[31] Employers may not discipline striking employees for merely participating in legal strikes.

In *Metropolitan Edison Company* v. *NLRB*,[32] the Supreme Court found that severe discipline imposed by management on union delegates for activity (or lack of it) in attempting to end a strike was unlawful under section 8(a)(3) of the NLRA. The Supreme Court did suggest, however, that an employer could negotiate into its collective bargaining agreement with the union specific actions that must be taken by union representatives during unlawful strikes.

In *Price Brothers Company*,[33] eight employees protested their discharge, which resulted from their participation in a wildcat strike. In this case, the arbitrator upheld the discharges, despite the fact that the employer merely believed the grievants to be guilty of a higher level of participation than other employees. The arbitrator ruled that the employer did not have to prove any greater degree of participation by the grievants. He reasoned that the employer acted in good faith:

> In the opinion of the arbitrator, it is not incumbent upon the Company to prove that the grievant participated in the strike to a greater degree than the other strikers before it can impose discipline upon him and not upon other strikers. The only obligation that the Company must meet is to show that it acted fairly and in good faith in arriving at its decision to discharge the grievant. The fact that its decision might be incorrect is irrelevant.
>
> When the grievant engaged in the wildcat strike, he subjected himself to the penalty of discharge. This penalty was prescribed by the Plant Rules and is a reasonable penalty for the offense involved. Likewise, the other strikers subjected themselves to the same penalty. The fact that the Company had a right to impose the penalty does not require it to do so. If it sees that it can invoke a lesser penalty or none at all, provided, however, that in making its decision as to who will be penalized it acts fairly and in good faith.

In *Avco Wyoming Division*,[34] the arbitrator upheld the company's selective discharge despite the absence of specific reference to discipline in the contract's no-strike clause, reasoning that "it would be an unconscionable denial of justice to 'tinker' with the discipline assessed. . . . The company is not obligated to denude its working force by wholesale discharges in order to preserve the validity of its no-strike agreement. It is not required to achieve a rigid, mechanical uniformity of treatment to a mathematical certainty; rather it is entitled to single out those more culpable and to be selective."

Some arbitrators have ruled differently, however. In *Superior Switchboard and Service Division*,[35] an arbitrator reinstated five workers who were discharged for organizing an illegal strike. He reasoned that disciplinary action was not specified in the contract's no-strike clause and in addition, management did not warn the individuals that they could or would be discharged for their actions. In this case, management not only failed to inform the individuals of possible disciplinary action but also "stood or sat idly by while employees around them argued about walking out, and some supervisors even actively encouraged the walkout."[36]

In *Payne & Keller, Inc.*,[37] the arbitrator reinstated an employee discharged for inciting a walkout. Here the arbitrator found that the individual making the accusations against the grievant was an unreliable witness and that there was no indication of actual job desertion.[38]

As indicated earlier, discipline may be imposed for employee misconduct during a legal strike. Examples of such misconduct are taunting strikebreakers, vandalism, and assaulting supervisors or others. The *Grievance Guide* published by the Bureau of National Affairs (BNA) has outlined the following criteria for discipline during a legal strike based on statements made by several arbitrators:[39]

- What is the extent of participation? In any mob situation, the degree of involvement of the individual in any action is important.

- What was the nature of the violence? This has both quantitative and qualitative aspects. Participation in several incidents is more serious than participation in only one. Some actions are more reprehensible than others. Shouting insults and shoving are of a different order from striking a person.

- Was the violence provoked? To the extent that the violence is retaliatory and defensive, it is less culpable than if undertaken as an act of aggression.

- Was the violence premeditated or undertaken on the spur of the moment? Premeditated violence is more inexcusable.

- What will be the impact of the punishment? Discharge is more of a penalty for an old man than a young one, for a long-service employee than a short-service employee.

- Was the disciplinary action discriminatory? A company is under some obligation to treat persons similarly situated in a comparable, although not necessarily identical, manner. Violence can hardly be said to be the real basis for discharge if other unjustifiable factors enter in.

- How serious was the offense in terms of injury to persons or damage to property?

- Were remedies at law available, and were they involved?

- Was the conduct destructive of good employee-employer relations?

- Was the conduct destructive of good community relations?

- Will the discipline restore good relations, or is it the result of a spirit of vindictiveness?

- Was the conduct such that the employee could be reabsorbed into the workforce?

Arbitrators have generally held that discipline less severe than discharge be imposed on employees for strike-related offenses committed after a strike ends. They reason that such offenses are emotionally generated.[40] An example is an offense of one union employee active in the strike against another who did not participate.

The following language is suggested for collective bargaining agreement no-strike or lockout sections to alleviate problems with employees who violate no-strike provisions: "The Employer shall have the right to discharge, with loss of all rights and benefits, or otherwise discipline any Employee who violates any provisions of the Article (and such discipline need not be uniform) and, in the event of a grievance is filed, the sole question for arbitration shall be whether the Employee engaged in prohibited activity."

In general, the end of a strike triggers temporary feelings of bitterness, pride, and frustration. Returning strike-supporting employees might harbor feelings of ill will against management, union employees who did not support the strike, and striker replacements. Their pent-up emotions are easily transformed into acts of misconduct.[41] The case of *Chromalloy American Corporation*[42] provides an example. In this case, an employee, upon returning to work after participating in a six-month strike, harassed workers hired as striker replacements, first through name-calling, labeling them "scabs," and later through actual threats to their safety and well-being. The employee was counseled for these actions and was finally terminated when he reported to work wearing a T-shirt imprinted with an obscene caption directed toward the replacement employees. The arbitrator reduced the termination to a suspension. The prior counseling, the arbitration said, was not sufficient because the employee had not been specifically warned that he would be terminated if he continued the misconduct.[43]

Resignation from the Union

Union employees who work during a strike can be subject to fines and other disciplinary action by the union. Employees can avoid this disciplinary action by resigning their union membership. Two sections of the NLRA support the employee's right to resign. Section 8b(l)(A), 29 U.S.C. Sec. 158 (b)(1)(A), provides:

> It shall be an unfair labor practice for a labor organization or its agents (1) to restrain or coerce … employees in the exercise of the rights guaranteed in Section 7. Provided, that this paragraph shall not impair the right of a labor organization to prescribe its own rules with respect to the acquisition or retention of membership therein.

Section 7, 29 U.S.C. Sec. 157, provides:

> Employees shall have the right to self-organization, to form, join, or assist labor organizations, to bargain collectively through representatives of their own choosing, and to engage in other concerted activities for the purpose of collective bargaining or other mutual aid or protection, and shall also have the right to refrain from any or all of such activities except to the extent that such right may be affected by an agreement requiring membership in a labor organization as a condition of employment as authorized in section 8(a)(3).

The Supreme Court ruled in *NLRB Granite State Joint Board, Textile Workers Union of America, Local 1029, AFL-CIO (International Paper Box Machine Company)*[44] and in *Booster Lodge No. 405, International Association of Machinists and Aerospace Workers, AFL-CIO (Boeing Company)* v. *NLRB*[45] that any attempt by the unions in these cases to fine former members for crossing an authorized picket line violated section 8(b)(1)(A) of the NLRA because the unions' constitutions and bylaws contained no provisions restricting members' rights to tender resignation.

In *Pattern Makers* v. *NLRB*,[46] the union's constitution prohibited resignations from the union during strikes. The Supreme Court in deciding the case determined that this was in violation of 8(b)(1)(A) of the NLRA, which makes it an unfair labor practice for a union to restrain or coerce employees in the exercise of their section 7 rights to self-organization. An employee, therefore, has the right to resign from a union at any time irrespective of any prohibitions that may exist in the union's constitution.

Any union member considering resignation from a union should send a letter of resignation, return receipt requested, to the union and should clearly indicate the effective date of that resignation.

Notes

1. Edwin F. Beal, Edward D. Wickersham, and Philip K. Keenest, *The Practice of Collective Bargaining,* 5th ed. (Homewood, Ill.: Irwin, 1976), pp. 19–20.

2. Beal, Wickersham, and Keenest, *The Practice of Collective Bargaining,* p. 20.

3. William K. Simkin, *Mediation and the Dynamics of Collective Bargaining* (Washington, D.C.: Bureau of National Affairs, 1971), p. 159.

4. Simkin, *Mediation,* p. 160.

5. Simkin, *Mediation,* p. 160.

6. Nancy Connolly Fibish, "The Board of Inquiry: A New Dimension in Private Sector Health Care Collective Bargaining," in Norman Metzger (ed.), *Handbook of Health Care Human Resources Management* (Rockville, Md.: Aspen, 1981), p. 756.

7. Lucretia Dewey Tanner, Harriet Goldberg Weinstein, and Alice Lynn Ahmuty, *Impact of the 1974 Health Care Amendments to the NLRA on Collective Bargaining in the Health Care Industry* (Washington, D.C.: U.S. Department of Labor, 1979), pp. 323–324.

8. Orley Ashenfelter and George Johnson, "Bargaining Theory, Trade Unions and Industrial Strike Activity," *American Economics Review,* Mar. 1969, pp. 35–49; Michael Shaler, "Trade Unionism and Economic Analysis: The Case of Industrial Conflict," *Journal of Labor Research,* Spring 1980, pp. 133–174; Bruce E. Kaufman, "Bargaining Theory, Inflation and Cyclical Strike Activity in Manufacturing," *Industrial and Labor Relations Review,* Apr. 1981, pp. 333–355; Bruce E. Kaufman, "The Determinants of Strikes in the United States, 1900–1977," *Industrial and Labor Relations Review,* July 1982.

9. Bruce E. Kaufman, "The Determinants of Strikes over Time and Across Industries," *Journal of Labor Research,* Spring 1983, p. 161.

10. Ashenfelter and Johnson, "Bargaining Theory"; Kaufman, "Bargaining Theory"; Kaufman, "Determinants of Strikes in the United States"; William J. Moore and Douglas K. Pearce, "A Comparative Analysis of Strike Models During Periods of Rapid Inflation, 1966–1977," *Journal of Labor Research,* Winter 1982, pp. 39–54.

11. Kaufman, "Determinants of Strikes over Time," p. 161.

12. Robert Wallace, "Factors Affecting Strike Decisions," unpublished Ph.D. dissertation, New School for Social Research, 1972; Robert N. Stern, "Intermetropolitan Patterns of Strike Frequency," *Industrial and Labor Relations Review,* Jan. 1976, pp. 218–235.

13. Kaufman, "Determination of Strikes over Time," p. 164.

14. Clark Kerr and Abraham Siegal, "The Interindustry Propensity to Strike," in Arthur Kornhauser, Robert Dubin, and Arthur Ross (eds.), *Industrial Conflict* (New York: McGraw-Hill, 1954), pp. 189–212.

15. Kaufman, "Determination of Strikes over Time," p. 165.

16. Paul E. Brody and Joseph B. Stamm, "Strike Two: Hospitals Down but Not Out," in Norman Metzger (ed.), *Handbook of Health Care Human Resources Management* (Rockville, Md.: Aspen, 1981), p. 760.

17. *Williams v. Pacific Marine Corporation*, 384 F.2d 935 (9th Cir. 1967), CA 1970; *Jersey Farms Milk Service, Inc., v. Meat Cutlers*, Cir. 4877 (M.D. Tenn. Jan. 16, 1969); *Navajo Freight Lines, Inc., v. Teamsters*, Civ. C-693 (D.C. Colo. October 18, 1968).

18. Bureau of National Affairs, *Grievance Guide,* 6th ed. (Washington, D.C.: Bureau of National Affairs, 1982), p. 285.

19. Bureau of National Affairs, *Grievance Guide*, p. 286.

20. *Fortex Manufacturing Company, Inc., v. Local 1065, Amalgamated Clothing and Textile Workers of America*, 76-2 ARB 8594.

21. *Foster Grading Company*, 52 LA 197.

22. Bureau of National Affairs, *Grievance Guide*, pp. 316–317.

23. Tanner, Weinstein, and Ahmuty, *Impact of the 1974 Health Care Amendments*, pp. 94–96.

24. Tanner, Weinstein, and Ahmuty, *Impact of the 1974 Health Care Amendments*, p. 73.

25. Tanner, Weinstein, and Ahmuty, *Impact of the 1974 Health Care Amendments*, p. 99.

26. *District 1199, National Union of Hospital and Health Care Employees Constitution*, p. 39.

27. Tanner, Weinstein, and Ahmuty, *Impact of the 1974 Health Care Amendments*, p. 94.

28. Tanner, Weinstein, and Ahmuty, *Impact of the 1974 Health Care Amendments*, p. 73.

29. Tanner, Weinstein, and Ahmuty, *Impact of the 1974 Health Care Amendments*, p. 99.

30. Bureau of National Affairs, *Grievance Guide*, p. 111.

31. Bureau of National Affairs, *Grievance Guide*, p. 111.

32. *Metropolitan Edison Company v. NLRB*, 663 F.2d 478, 108 LRRM 3020 (CA 3, 1981).

33. *Price Brothers Company*, 74 LA 748.

34. *Avco Wyoming Division*, 51 LA 1228.

35. *Superior Switchboard and Service Division*, 75 LA 1107.

36. Bureau of National Affairs, *Grievance Guide*, pp. 114–115.

37. *Payne & Keller, Inc.*, 70 LA 114.

38. Bureau of National Affairs, *Grievance Guide*, p. 115.

39. Bureau of National Affairs, *Grievance Guide*, p. 116.

40. Bureau of National Affairs, *Grievance Guide*, p. 118.

41. Bureau of National Affairs, *Grievance Guide*, p. 118.

42. *Chromalloy American Corporation*, 72 LA 8383.

43. Bureau of National Affairs, *Grievance Guide*, p. 118.

44. *NLRB Granite State Joint Board, Textile Workers Union of America, Local 1029, AFL-CIO (International Paper Box Machine Company)*, 109 U.S. 213 (1972).

45. *Booster Lodge No. 405, International Association of Machinists and Aerospace Workers, AFL-CIO (Boeing Company)* v. *NLRB*, 412 U.S. 84 (1973).

46. *Pattern Makers* v. *NLRB*, 473 U.S. 95 (1985).

Chapter 4

Nursing Strikes

A Breed Apart

WHEN ATTEMPTING to distinguish strikes by nurses from those by service, maintenance, technical, clerical, security, and other nonmedical employees in the health care industry, the following guideposts help:

- Significant differences exist between these employee groups in relation to the role each plays in the overall delivery of patient care as perceived by the employees, hospital administration, the public, and above all, the patient.

- All the groups share common concerns for security and recognition.

- Notwithstanding the meeting ground of needs, professional nurses have established themselves as a separate and unique bargaining unit.

The functions of all employees within a health care facility are obviously important to the facility's effective operation. Patient care is a team responsibility. Any walkout can pose administrative and patient care dilemmas. Nevertheless, some groups represent more of a threat than others. The key here, of course, is the extent to which a health care facility can adequately continue to provide "hands-on" patient care services during such work stoppages.

When District 1199, National Union of Hospital and Health Care Employees, struck New York City hospitals and nursing homes in 1976 and 1984, the hospitals and homes continued to operate, albeit at different levels of occupancy, throughout the strikes' respective eleven- and forty-seven-day durations. Employing strike contingency plans, the hospitals and homes continued operations at near-normal levels, utilizing the services of supervisors, volunteers, temporary or agency employees, and professional employees. These nonstriking employees worked virtually around the clock and maintained patient care operations. An earlier strike—in November

1973—by District 1199 against the same hospitals and homes, though of shorter duration, had a more negative effect on the delivery of patient care. In that strike, both the Committee of Interns and Residents and the New York State Nurses Association actively sympathized with the strikers and instructed their members to perform only the duties of their classifications.[1]

In contrast to strikes by nonnursing personnel, a nursing strike requires an available source of temporary registered nurses along with nonunion nursing personnel if the facility is to remain operational. This was clearly demonstrated during the New York State Nurses Association strike at Maimonides Hospital in Brooklyn from March 30 through April 18, 1998, during which the hospital remained almost fully operational with an infusion of temporary nursing staff working twelve-hour shifts. Nursing strikes in which temporary employees are not utilized or available inevitably result in curtailed services and patient census.

The critical importance to patient care of the attending physician and the house staff is readily recognized. Too often the role of the nurse is less appreciated. Professional nurses contribute significantly to patient care. They play an unusual role in the patient care family—more equal than others and therefore more essential. City and state health codes mandate a nurse's presence in many phases and areas of patient care. New York City health codes, for instance, require that a circulating nurse be present in an operating room where cesarean section deliveries are performed and that at least one registered nurse be on staff for every ten maternity patients on day shifts and every twenty patients on other shifts. No less important is the matter of patient perception. Many patients view nurses as more important to their total recuperation process than their own attending physicians. Hospital patients recognize the essential role that physicians play, but patients see their doctors only periodically. In contrast, the nurse is by the patient's side daily, comforting and assisting the patient's recovery.

A human resource administrator of an institution that experienced a nursing walkout lasting ninety-eight days stated, "One of our major considerations from the strike's very beginning was assuring the remaining patient population (those who could not be discharged or relocated) that care would continue to be provided by physicians, supervisory nurses, replacement nurses, LPNs, and aides. " He added that "patient fear, for the most part, centered on a loss of personalized daily health care services provided by the nurse who, to the patient, was always there." Patients generally do not recognize the contribution of the other very dedicated and hardworking but often unseen employees, such as porters, painters, aides, food service workers, guards, or clerks. Patients perceive the nurse as the primary provider of care and comfort during their time of need. An antediluvian image of "angels of mercy" still exists. This phenomenon is widely known as "Nightingalism," so named for the nineteenth-century health crusader Florence Nightingale. Strictly interpreted, Nightingalism is self-sacrifice, service given without concern for economic reward or job conditions.[2] Notwithstanding the outdated nature of such a perception, it is one of the important factors that distinguishes strikes by nurses from those by other employee groups. Present in most nurse confrontations with health care institutions are the pressures on nurses not to abandon their patients, pressure on the hospital administrator to act responsibly to avoid such walkouts, and the lack of understanding and therefore lack of support of such action by the patients and the public.

A Series of Conflicts

Obvious conflicts exist in perceptions of what nurses are or should be, how they should conduct themselves professionally while attempting to improve their working conditions and wages, and the extent to which nurses should act collectively to control their own destiny. These conflicts weave the intricately complex web of irony and agony that ensnares nurses, patients, hospital administrators, unions, and the public.

There are people who contend, despite the myriad of published studies, surveys, and analyses highlighting the nurses' frustration over denial of true professional status, that it is the nurse who practices sophistry. To these skeptics, nurses are ambivalent; they cannot make up their minds as to whether they wish to be recognized as health care professionals or as unionists (the skeptics perceive an inherent conflict between the two). Is this an antilabor philosophy? Not necessarily; some union leaders share this view. They see unions as having played an important role in the shaping of wages and conditions for the traditional (blue-collar) worker, but they contend that a nurse is a professional, not a worker. The case for such differentiation is unfounded. The dictionary defines a profession as a "field of endeavor in which individuals are engaged for gain; and . . . engaged in by persons receiving financial return." Further, professionalism is "the following of a profession for gain or livelihood." There exists a definite relationship between professionals and other workers, as well as a common interest in bettering working conditions, which has driven professionals to unionize.

Other analysts profess that the unionization of nurses is acceptable and understandable. The use of the strike, or even the threat of a strike, is, however, seriously questioned as a "professional" option. But how effective is the collective bargaining process without the threat of a strike? Michael

Miller states that "when the negotiation process is unsuccessful, the parties involved may be forced to use their relative economic strength. For the health care facility this means using its ability to withstand a strike. For the staff it means the ability to withstand forced unemployment. For the patients it may mean uncertain health care. Nevertheless, the use of economic strength may be the only means, although not necessarily the desirable means, of achieving bargaining or other objectives."[3]

This kind of thinking generated the withdrawal of the no-strike policy by the American Nurses Association (ANA) at its national convention in 1968. Established in 1950, the no-strike pledge, for all of its eighteen-year existence, conflicted with the association's ability to conduct effective collective bargaining with health care employers. Barbara G. Shutt, editor of the *American Journal of Nursing,* stated in a 1968 article that the no-strike policy "assumes that employers would demonstrate, on their part, a sense of obligation and good will by dealing with the nurses' representatives. With a few sterling exceptions, nurses' employers proved to be as unwilling as most other employers to negotiate with employee groups."[4]

Early Objectives and Changing Directions

Prior to World War II, the ANA engaged in an economic security program; however, the policy of the program did not include collective bargaining. Although nurses' strikes and concerted efforts had occurred, the national organization did not sanction them.[5] Organized in 1896, the association's stated main purposes were as follows:[6]

1. To establish and maintain a code of ethics
2. To elevate the standards of nursing education
3. To promote the financial and other interests of the nursing profession

In this third purpose lay the roots of conflict that would surface seventy-two years later. In a pioneering position, the ANA stated that the nurses should not "seriously consider forming or participating in organizations which accept as a principle 'a collective withdrawal from work' even as a 'last resort.'"[7] Apparently, the association founders did not comprehend the incongruity of attempting to the promote financial interests of its members while forbidding those same members to join organizations that might exercise economic pressures to achieve such objectives.

The California Nurses Association (CNA) has been an innovator in protecting and improving the economic conditions of nurses.[8] In 1966, two years prior to similar action by the national association, the CNA rescinded its no-strike policy. In 1943, after securing a 15 percent salary increase from the National War Labor Board, the CNA implemented a total economic security program and signed its first contract with the San Francisco Bay Area hospitals in 1946.[9] Its success, the acceleration of union organizing, and the persistent low level of nurse compensation led the ANA in 1946 to adopt an economic security program, including collective bargaining.[10] It issued the following policy statement: "The American Nurses Association believes that the several state and district nurses associations are qualified to act and should act as the exclusive agents of their respective memberships in the important fields of economic security and collective bargaining. The Association . . . urges all state and district nurses associations to push such a program vigorously and expeditiously."[11]

By 1948, nurses associations in Washington, Minnesota, and Oregon had also been recognized as bargaining agents for their members, and in the same year, twenty-two state associations adopted the ANA economic security program.[12] By 1961, associations in forty-eight of the fifty states had adopted the program.

When the ANA adopted the no-strike policy in 1950, it also adopted a neutrality policy (which remained effective until 1970) in disputes that did not involve nurses.[13] The neutrality policy recommended that nurses remain neutral in conflicts involving other employee groups and that nurses not perform tasks outside their normal duties. The ANA reissued its policy subsequent to strikes throughout the country in 1958 and 1959.[14] The no-strike pledge was adopted in anticipation that as a quid pro quo for the continuation of work guarantee, the association would expect good faith collective bargaining from health care employers.

Unfortunately for nurses, collective bargaining was not the panacea for their problems. Even with mediation and fact-finding panels, nurses found many of their goals unrealized in the collective bargaining process. Without a measure of force—which was still banned by the ANA's no-strike policy—most nurses saw little chance of making major breakthroughs toward their objectives. Some claimed that employers abstained from meaningful give-and-take negotiations and adhered to whatever criteria they deemed reasonable.[15]

The 1950s and early 1960s proved frustrating to nurses. Many felt a sense of impotence in the collective bargaining arena. Prior to the rescission of the no-strike pledge by the CNA in 1966, the festering frustration began to push nurses into collective work action, and nurse employee groups emerged as formidable collective bargaining adversaries. From this time on, nurses harnessed and wielded power on a national level. The nightmare of nurses abandoning their patients turned into a stark reality. Nurses went out on strike in distressingly large numbers. The shock waves resounded throughout the health care industry.

In 1961, mass nurse resignations developed as a tool for realizing gains. In April of that year, the Illinois Nursing Association was refused a meeting with the administration of Keewanee Hospital, a voluntary not-for-profit hospital; the nurses turned in their resignations. Nurses at eight hospitals in Orange County, California, also resigned en masse to demonstrate for recognition.[16] During the mid-1960s, the use of mass resignation and picketing increased substantially. Nurses became aggressive in their demands and enforced them by strikes, sick-outs, and mass resignations. These actions occurred in San Francisco, New York City, and Los Angeles, among other areas.[17] After thirteen days, nurses in Youngstown, Ohio, returned to work, having won a 19 percent raise.[18] In hospitals in other major cities, nurse resignations brought managements close to total submission to the demonstrating nurses' demands for improved benefits. In effect, resignation was achieving the same results as a strike.

Why did the nurses prefer resignation to strikes? There was still the matter of the ANA's no-strike pledge, and more important, at that time nurses still believed that it was wrong to abandon their commitment to the patient by conducting job actions and picketing. They perceived this approach as unprofessional. Resignation was a means to an end "with honor." The nurses would, with a minimum amount of guilt, leave the hospital, or the profession for that matter, to eliminate the stress they were experiencing. They were not betraying their professional vows. They were merely "getting out of a bad situation." As Michael Miller points out, "Employees who hand in their resignations supposedly have no intention of returning to their jobs even if changes are made; . . . resignation concerns the right of individuals to work for the employer they wish and under the circumstances they prefer. Although the philosophy of mass resignation and [that of] striking are different . . . mass resignation functions in the same manner as a strike."[19]

The nurses did not want to resign their positions. They were frustrated and out of a sense of guilt could not indulge in a strike. Then the idea of a job action as a means of achieving desired working condition improvements began to be openly discussed and considered as an alternative to resignation. Nurses reasoned that although it might be considered unprofessional to walk out on patients, doing so might be the only effective means available to obtain changes, and further, such action would ultimately redound to the benefit of patient care.

Barbara Shutt's appointment in 1960 to the editorship of the *American Journal of Nursing* significantly boosted the collective action movement of nurses. Her appointment gave the economic security program a national platform. She used the journal to communicate to the nation's nurses, frequently and militantly. Prior to 1960, only about three thousand nurses worked under ANA-negotiated contracts. By the end of 1960, approximately eighteen thousand nurses—a 700 percent increase—were under contract.[20]

No-Strike Pledge Rescinded

In its no-strike policy rescission statement, the ANA supported "the efforts of the State Nurses Associations acting as bargaining representatives for members in taking necessary steps to achieve improved conditions, including use of concerted economic pressures which are lawful and consistent with the nurses' professional responsibilities and with the public need."[21] Shutt lauded the policy reversal and stated in the journal, "After eighteen agonizing and economically almost fruitless years, it finally became clear that the policy was unrealistic, practically unenforceable and at best misleading, if not dishonest."[22] The die was cast! The conflict resolved! Collective bargaining in the health care industry would never be quite the same.

In 1969, two noteworthy strikes occurred, one in Los Angeles and the other in San Francisco. The strikes are noteworthy because of the issue common to both. Both strikes, which collectively lasted sixty-two days, resulted in settlements that granted a demand aimed at improving deteriorating staffing conditions—the creation of the Professional Practice Committee. Common in nursing contracts today, the Professional Practice Committee provided for a joint-committee composition of members of management and nursing staff, which would meet periodically to discuss development of staffing patterns, problems in patient care, and existing conflict situations between physicians and nurses. These "noneconomic demands," seen by many hospital administrators as erosive of management rights, would become common in the years that followed.

The Calm Before the Storm

The early 1970s were essentially quiet years, but the atmosphere was to change. If we were to consider this period the calm before the storm, the atmospheric disturbance to come would be manifest in two major events: first, the twenty-one-day strike by the CNA against hospitals and clinics in the San Francisco Bay Area in 1974, and second, Public Law 93-360, effective August 25, 1974, which amended the National Labor Relations Act (NLRA) and repealed the exemption that had been incorporated into the act in 1947.[23] Under the 1974 amendments, the same rights and privileges would now be granted to all not-for-profit hospital workers—numbering 1.6 million and employed in 3,400 institutions—as had been legislated for most other workers thirty-nine years earlier. The 1974 amendments intensified union activity among nurses, and by the early 1980s, the number of ANA member nurses working under bargaining contracts had risen to about eighty thousand, a more-than-fourfold increase since 1960.

On June 7, 1974, approximately 4,400 registered nurses struck forty-one hospitals and clinics in the San Francisco Bay Area. Although the CNA, which represented the nurses, sought economic gains inclusive of pension improvements, its main demand was for a voice in staffing pattern decisions. During its annual convention in San Francisco, the CNA House of Delegates, while soliciting support from its member attendees, resolved to establish a special fund that would assist its striking members. The crippled hospitals submitted to almost all of the CNA's demands, ending the twenty-one-day-old strike. The nurses achieved two major inroads into patient care decision making:[24]

1. Registered nurses (RNs) have a right to take part in determining how many nurses are needed for intensive care, renal dialysis, postanesthesia recovery, and other nursing units. Boards of directors composed solely of doctors and hospital administrators cannot make decisions on staffing these units without input from knowledgeable nurses.

2. The hospital boards must establish procedures so that nurses can advise on staffing needs for medical-surgical and other patients requiring special nursing care. Hospitals will pay the nurses for participation on these professional performance committees.

On July 12, 1976, approximately eighteen hundred nurses struck fifteen hospitals in and around Seattle, Washington. Area newspapers defined the issues as demands for RN input into patient care, ongoing in-service education, limited shift rotation, mandatory Washington State Nurses Association (WSNA) membership, a cost-of-living salary increase, recognition of the increased complexity of patient care, and a shift differential.[25] The strike lasted approximately sixty-eight days, cutting patient population by 50 percent during that time.

In 1997 and 1998, the California Nurses Association staged five one- and two-day strikes involving 7,500 Kaiser Permanente nurses at approximately fifty hospitals and clinics throughout Northern California. Clearly, the hesitancy to use strikes as a weapon has been significantly diminished.

A Breed Apart

One group of researchers determined that "in collective bargaining, the nurses' definition of a situation might be quite different from that of health service management; thus, their reasons for striking and their assessment of the bargaining issues would not be congruent with those of management."[26] While many hospital administrators feel that industrial sector bargaining issues, such as wages and job security, are critical problems for nurses, in reality the nurses are more concerned about communication with management and participation in organizational decision making. In fact, these last two issues have important implications in their impact on predicting strike behavior. Again and again, studies point out that an overwhelmingly large number of nurses have concerns quite different from those of other employees, and these concerns spill over into collective bargaining. The following concerns are foremost among nurses:

- The inability to communicate concerns to management

- Authoritarian behavior on the part of management

- Understaffing

- Lack of respect from physicians

- Lack of control over nursing practice

- Lack of support from nursing administration

- Dissatisfaction with shift assignments, floating rotations, weekend scheduling, and mandatory overtime

A marked difference between traditional collective bargaining and collective bargaining with nurses is the ability to take "several bites of the apple." It is a hallowed concept of traditional collective bargaining that management makes the deal at the bargaining table, that all issues are aired, and that a settlement, once arrived at, concludes the bargain. This is not always true with professional groups. Because of market pressures, nursing shortages, and turnover, midyear, midcontract adjustments are not unusual.

The Taft-Hartley Act requires the parties to bargain about "wages, hours, and other terms and conditions of employment." These are the traditional issues addressed at the collective bargaining table. They may not always be amenable to early settlement, but the process of collective bargaining has proved to be well suited to their resolution. With nurses, a variety of other issues complicate the bargain. Shortly after the Health Care Amendments to the act, an article appeared in the *American Journal of Nursing* that stated: "The jurisdictional expansion of the NLRA to include employees of private health care institutions can become an opportunity for the nursing profession to increase its influence and control over the practice of nursing. The labor contract . . . becomes a legal instrument *through* which the profession can implement standards of care. . . . Collective bargaining can be an effective process for bringing about a redistribution of the base of power within the health service organization."[27]

This analysis proved to be a self-fulfilling prophecy. Such an interpretation pervaded nursing associations, which organized RNs in the years following the passage of the amendments.

Nurses seek shared governance, that is, a role in shaping rights and responsibilities to determine the nature of the delivery and quality of patient care. Such issues have proved extremely difficult to resolve in the collective bargaining arena. Institutions usually do not have the resources to resolve these concerns, and the parties sometimes, in the end, seek resolution through legal channels. However, as most experienced labor relations practitioners know, few contracts are resolved and few strikes surrendered as a result of legal decisions.

The Bargaining Process

Collective bargaining with nurses has proved to be extremely complex and fraught with the danger of impasse and ensuing strikes. The frustrations expressed by Candice Owley, chair of the Federation of Nurses and Health Professions of the American Federation of Teachers–United Federation of Teachers, at a seminar on collective bargaining are exemplary. She explained why nurses are angry: "We don't like our working conditions, we don't like the image that is portrayed, and we don't like each other, and we don't like the doctors. . . ." Such frustrations are common and are often brought to the bargaining table with growing militancy, chaos, and ill will. Strikes result. In such situations, the community is at risk.

It is not only the nurses who are frustrated within the collective bargaining process. Often management participants find the difference between traditional bargaining and nurse bargaining frustrating and difficult to handle. Settlements are hammered out only to be rejected quickly by rank-and-file nurses. The immediate analysis of management is that units represented by nursing associations are often uncontrollable. A knee-jerk management condemnation of the leadership of nurses' associations follows, but when clearer heads look around, they find a similar rejection of settlements by units represented by traditional trade unions. It is clear that even given the most skilled labor negotiators and the best of intentions on both sides, settlement rejections can still proliferate and strikes can still result. The commitments made on and off the record by union representatives have frittered away in the face of rank-and-file rejection. These votes of "no confidence" in their union leadership reflect a broader problem than individual rejection. This inability of nurse union leaders to translate the real concerns of nurses into acceptable settlements has played a role in the proliferation of strikes by professional nurses.

Anatomy of Three Nursing Strikes

Several years ago, three separate bargaining units at three separate hospitals, made up of several thousand professional nurses, reached bargaining impasses and went out on strike.

Upon receiving the ten-day strike notice, the first institution immediately curtailed occupancy. It halted elected admissions, and doctors examined their patients by service, recommending, where appropriate, discharge or transfer. This strike lasted five full days. Occupancy rates declined from an average of 92 percent to 25 percent. The institution did not lay off any other employees, union or nonunion. Nonunion registered nurses (nurse supervisors and administrative nurses), LPNs, aides, and house staff provided nursing services. Some unionized nurses, even though part of the bargaining unit out on strike, came in to staff critical care areas. It took six full days after the strike to return to normal occupancy. The hospital lost an estimated $4 million. This hospital had a high ratio of RNs to LPNs and nursing aides.

Believing that the strike would last a day or two, the administrator of the second hospital decided not to curtail occupancy. When the strike ensued, nurse supervisors, LPNs, and aides provided the nursing services. The hospital did screen admissions to identify the more acutely ill patients. Some consolidation of units took place. On the third and last day of the strike, the hospital discharged many patients and cut back on admissions. However, curtailment of services never exceeded 20 percent. The financial impact of the strike was minimal. Interestingly, both the first and second hospitals have attempted since the strikes to hire more LPNs and have made concerted efforts to exclude head nurses from bargaining units.

The third hospital suffered a disastrous strike. It was one of the longest strikes on record at that time. One of the key issues was the union's position regarding floating. The hospital had a policy that provided for floating employees throughout the hospital. The union wanted this policy eliminated. During the strike, supervisors, clinical coordinators, head nurses, and assistant head nurses provided the nursing services. The hospital began to recruit per diems and full-time replacements. They sought assistance from private agencies and paid premium salaries to nurses who would cross the picket line to replace striking nurses. Occupancy, which had been 90 percent or higher before the strike, moved sharply downward to approximately 50 percent. Patients were discharged immediately after receipt of the ten-day strike notice. Elective admissions were discontinued. By the first week of the strike, only 300 of the hospital's 550 beds were occupied. By the third week of the strike, occupancy was at 225 beds. A total of 140 nurses provided services for these 225 patients.

Negotiations were suspended as soon as the strike occurred, and no meetings were scheduled for the first two weeks of the strike. Positions hardened. Negotiations began again in the third week. Federal mediation was involved, but a board of inquiry was not appointed because both parties rejected the idea. The union brought new issues to the table once negotiations resumed, and issues that had been withdrawn by the union in negotiations prior to the strike were reintroduced. Positions hardened further. A settlement was fashioned, but the membership overwhelmingly rejected it. Once again the ugly difference in nurse negotiations reared its head: the negotiating group did not speak for the membership.

Negotiations floundered. The hospital continued to operate with only 225 beds occupied. Because no other group of employees at the hospital was organized, the hospital did not lay off anyone, hoping that its nonunionized employees would see this effort at saving their jobs as a symbol. Financial losses were staggering, and pressure was placed on the hospital to settle. After one of the longest nursing strikes on record at that time, a settlement was hammered out and overwhelmingly approved.

The hospital lost more than $1 million. It took more than a month after the strike ended to get back to the original occupancy in excess of 90 percent. The returning nurses were extremely militant. As one hospital administrator pointed out, "We went through an earthquake, and we are now feeling the aftershock." The hospital agreed to bring all the striking nurses back, but it also retained any new nurses hired during the strike. Antagonism between the two groups was high, and grievances increased.

Strike Impact

Nursing strikes are different from other strikes. Their impact is dramatically greater than strikes by nonnurses. The issues are often complex and less amenable to settlement across the collective bargaining table. Whether legally mandatory items for bargaining or not, the issues are put on the table and become threshold issues, frequently blocking settlements. Bargaining leadership is often permissive and unable to reflect the real concerns of the bargaining unit and, more often, unwilling to exercise control. Salary source replacements for strikers are readily available, a fact that further sets nurses apart from other labor groups.

Notes

1. League of Voluntary Hospitals and Homes of New York, *Hospital Strike* (New York: League of Voluntary Hospitals and Homes of New York, 1973), p. 1.

2. Norma K. Grand, "Nightingalism, Employeeism, and Professional Collectivism," *Nursing Forum*, 1971, *10*, 289.

3. Michael H. Miller, "Nurses' Right to Strike," *Journal of Nursing Administration*, 1975, *5*, 35–39.

4. Barbara G. Shutt, "The Right to Strike," *American Journal of Nursing*, 1968, *26*(10).

5. D. Wood, "They Live and Learn with Unions," *Modern Hospital*, 1959, *93*, 73–74.

6. G. J. Griffin and J. Griffin, *Jensen's History and Trends of Professional Nursing*, 6th ed. (St. Louis, Mo.: Mosby, 1969), p. 116.

7. "Nurses' Unions?" *American Journal of Nursing*, 1968, *36*, 1122.

8. Norman Metzger and Dennis D. Pointer, *Labor-Management Relations in the Health Services Industry: Theory and Practice* (Washington, D.C.: Science and Health Publications, 1972), p. 37.

9. Ronald L. Miller, "Development and Structure of Collective Bargaining Among Registered Nurses," *Personnel Journal*, 1971, *5*, 134.

10. Lyndia Flanagan, *One Strong Voice: The Story of the American Nurses Association* (Kansas City, Mo.: American Nurses Association, 1976), p. 168.

11. American Nurses Association, *Major Official Policies Relating to the Economic Security Program* (New York: American Nurses Association, 1965), p. 1.

12. American Nurses Association, "The Economic Security Program," *American Journal of Nursing*, 1947, *47*, 190.

13. J. Seidman, "Nurses and Collective Bargaining," *Industrial and Labor Relations Reviews*, 1970, *23*, 342.

14. American Nurses Association, "If a Hospital Strike Occurs," *American Journal of Nursing*, 1960, *60*, 344–347.

15. Miller, "Nurses' Right to Strike," p. 35.

16. Metzger and Pointer, *Labor-Management Relations*, p. 36.

17. Dorothy Peters, "The Keewanee Story," *American Journal of Nursing*, 1961, *61*(10), 74–79.

18. "Youngstown Nurses End Thirteen-Day Walkout; Michigan Nurses Sign First Agreement," *White Collar Report*, 1966, *74*(5), 1.

19. Miller, "Nurses' Right to Strike."

20. "Program Briefs," *American Journal of Nursing*, 1961, *61*(9), 74.

21. American Nurses Association, *ANA's Economic and General Welfare Program: Philosophy, Goals, Policies, Positions* (Kansas City, Mo.: American Nurses Association, 1976), p. 5.

22. Shutt, "The Right to Strike."

23. S. M. Kaynard, "Health Care Industry Under the National Labor Relations Act," in Norman Metzger (ed.), *Handbook of Health Care Human Resources Management* (Rockville, Md.: Aspen, 1981), p. 537.

24. "Nurses Set Precedent in Gains from San Francisco Strike," *RN,* Sept. 1974.

25. "Mini on the Scene; Seattle, Washington," *Nursing Administration Quarterly,* 1982, *6*(2), 41–58.

26. Joan R. Bloom, G. Nicholas Parlette, and Charles A. O'Reilly, "Collective Bargaining by Nurses: A Comparative Analysis of Management and Employee Perceptions," *Health Care Management Review,* 1980, *5*(1), 25–33.

27. Virginia Cleland, "The Professional Model," *American Journal of Nursing,* 1975, *75*(2), 288.

Chapter 5

The Future

Proposals for Change

THE TRADITIONAL VIEW subscribed to by both management and union practitioners as to the place of strikes in the collective bargaining arena was expressed by Bernard Karsh:

> The strike is among the most highly publicized and the least studied social phenomena of our time.... [It] is the mechanism which produces that increment of pressure necessary to force agreement where differences are persistent and do not yield to persuasion or argument around the bargaining table.... The alternate to such a system might result in the demise of the collective bargaining system as we know it; some form of coercion exercised by a supreme authority, whether it be a government board, an industrial relations court, compulsory arbitrations, or some other of the many proposals which have been advanced from time to time, would supplant the voluntarism implicit in the American collective bargaining experience. Thus, the strike, or threat of strike, is the ultimate device whereby the competing interests of antagonistic parties are expediently resolved, leading to a modus operandi which permits both sides to accommodate their differences and live with one another.[1]

In the health care industry as in other industries, strikes and strike threats are integral parts of the total industrial collective bargaining experience. It is not unusual for administrators of nonunion institutions to believe that union recognition is a direct invitation to strikes. Where contract terms are not settled to a union's satisfaction, strikes will be used to force management to compromise its position and meet the union's demands, either in full or in part. Labor law requires that management and labor bargain "in good faith," but it does not compel them to agree to proposals made by either side. Unions can and do strike to support their positions in negotiations. The strike is part of the arsenal of weapons available to the union, which intends to make it expensive and inconvenient for the employer not to agree to its proposals.[2]

The right to strike continues to be defended by many experts, but strife on the health care labor front and in other industrial areas, including the discomforting strikes of transit workers, teachers, police officers, firefighters, and other public sector employees, has raised a hue and cry among the public.[3] Public approval of stoppages wanes as unemployment rises and unemployed workers look askance at individuals who have the opportunity to work during economically depressed times but elect to withhold their services.

Some observers feel that health care unions, by striking, do not punish their employers but rather the patients and, of course, the public. That same public has now found that the strike, in seeking to apply pressure if not to cause injury to the employer, has many by-products that affect the broader community, including inconvenience and the passing along of higher costs for products or services to the public. Far more important is the awareness that the strike of health care workers may well be a threat to the continued uninterrupted delivery of lifesaving services.

The Effect of Strikes

The impact of any strike on consumers of the product involved is related to three considerations: the cultural necessity of the product, the stock effect, and the possibility of substitution.[4] "Cultural necessity" is defined as the importance of the product in the lives of the people who consume it. Products that are dispensable or deferrable may be considered unnecessary; other products must be available if hardship is to be avoided; and at the top of the scale, some products are necessary for health and safety.

The "stock effect" is the extent to which consumption declines as stocks diminish. In a milk strike, for example, as the stock of milk in the stores declines, the impact of the strike increases.

The third factor, the possibility of substituting other products for the "struck" products, ranges from a completely acceptable substitute at the lower end of the scale to the top of the scale, where no acceptable substitute is available.

A strike at a hospital or nursing home has a high impact. The end product, patient care, is absolutely necessary; this is not debatable. As to the stock effect, a strike removes beds from the available stock in the community, thus extending waiting lists, and mitigates the provision of emergency services.

Regarding the last factor, the lack of acceptable substitutes in most communities is quite apparent.

The real losers in strikes at health care institutions are the patients, their families, and prospective patients. The patients will be underserved, may be moved from the struck hospital or home, or may be discharged earlier than they should be. Families of patients will be subjected to anxieties over the limited care that is available and may be forced to administer home care. Prospective patients will be troubled by the limited available beds, operations will be delayed, and outpatient care will be discontinued.

Health Care Strikes: Are They Defensible?

The appropriateness of collective bargaining as it is now practiced in health care institutions is suspect. Are strikes, walkouts, or the threat of either of these traditional labor weapons necessary or acceptable when, in the final analysis, they directly or indirectly reduce the quality of patient care? Charles Darwin commented that he had steadily endeavored to keep his mind free so as to give up any hypothesis, however much beloved (and he further commented that he could not resist forming one on every subject), as soon as facts are shown to be opposed. The facts are, indeed, clearly opposed to the old hypothesis of the rationalization of the need for strikes in health care collective bargaining. The pendulum has swung in the health care industry from a minimal concern for employee relations to an almost distracting overemphasis on that area. Concern for employees is, of course, an essential part of quality health care. The unions have been instrumental in directing our focus on the needs of employees. But who represents the patients? Who speaks for the sick, the seriously ill, the concerned patients who need the full attention of our medical staff? What comfort is it to patients to know that a strike is threatened or that a walkout may take place when they are in desperate need of attention? How are the fears of the elderly allayed when the workers at a home for the aged walk out over contract negotiations?

Many practitioners point to the low incidence of strikes in our society, but the possibility of a strike or the threat of one remains a reality in the health care industry. In many areas, unions, nurtured by management and governmental representatives, have become masters of brinkmanship, which makes patients ill at ease. Someone once said that an industry gets the kind of labor relations it deserves. Do we in health care truly deserve the industrial model? Is confrontation necessary, or even permissible, where patient care is involved? Health care collective bargaining must be more than an adversarial relationship built on an aggression containment model. It must be more than a fistfight. Only children and incomplete adults think that life is a continuous test of strength and that one side must always prevail. D. Quinn Mills believes that managers and union officials must always have at the top of their agenda the broadening of cooperation and consensus.[5] We must attempt to move the collective bargaining process beyond continual confrontation and into a more constructive mode. Some new approaches should be developed to minimize crisis bargaining. Relationships should be altered. Management must be a partner in this review of alternative approaches to the present model. The unions, of course, should seek innovative remedies and take the lead in designing an equitable arbitration system that would settle the contract disputes of public and health care employees without destructive strikes.[6] Both unions and management must be willing to take a chance and pay the price. They have not been willing to do so in the past.

Alternatives to the Strike

The quest for impasse procedures that will make strikes unnecessary in the health care industry is a relatively new undertaking. Some health care labor contracts contain interest arbitration clauses that prohibit strikes, and some states have such provisions for public sector employees and have included health care employees within that jurisdiction, but such provisions and laws are generally opposed by both parties to the collective bargaining agreement. This is difficult to understand, for binding arbitration laws have been relatively successful in the public sector. Arguments against binding arbitration are mostly theoretical and are based on the premise of the chilling effect of such provisions on collective bargaining. Attempts to consider any mechanism that prohibits strikes in the health care industry have been stymied in the past for much the same reasons that such attempts have been stalled in the public sector. John Beamer points out that despite the relative success of binding arbitration laws, a large number of individuals are unable or unwilling to consider alternatives to the strike.[7] They support their opposition to binding arbitration with arguments from the past, positions taken before the laws were really tested, arguments that are, in essence, more fiction than fact. The health care industry can learn a great deal from the successful experiment with alternatives to strikes in public employment.

Impasse resolution methods include fact-finding, conventional interest arbitration, final-offer arbitration, and mediation-arbitration.

Fact-Finding

Fact-finding is a discipline quite different from mediation. The mediator often provides the parties with a method to communicate without face-to-face confrontations. The mediator is often both a messenger and a persuader. The mediator attempts to clarify arguments and channel the parties into positions of compromise. Fact finders, either in a panel or singularly, are responsible for establishing relevant facts in a dispute and often recommend compromise positions. Tripartite panels usually consist of a representative from the employer, one from the union, and a neutral representative selected jointly by both parties. A fact finder can be a single party as well. In either case, panel or individual, the fact finder is charged with developing the facts of the dispute through a hearing with, in some cases, the rights to subpoena and to render an opinion or to recommend a settlement of the dispute based on the acquired information.[8]

There are four types of fact-finding. The first is fact-finding without recommendations. A fact finder who is not empowered to give recommendations examines the events that have transpired and evaluates the areas of factual difference. This process is usually an exercise in futility because most labor disputes are so complicated that a mere portrayal of facts does not create the basis for a settlement.[9] The second type of fact finder also makes no recommendations. This kind of fact-finding takes place well in advance of the actual negotiations. In such cases, an impartial person or agency is appointed before negotiations have begun to develop a factual background for future use by the bargainers. For example, impartial actuaries or insurance experts can provide a single set of facts about the costs of a variety of hypothetical pension and insurance benefits. President Kennedy's Advisory Committee on Labor-Management Policy recommended this system in 1962. It normally precedes a stalemate and helps avoid a strike.[10]

Another type of fact-finding involves recommendations on procedures or direction without recommendations on issue. The Taylor-Higgins-Reedy Board used this method when handling the 1967–1968 disputes in the nonferrous metals industry. During the negotiations, the parties were stalemated over a demand by the union for coordinated bargaining. The board did not attempt to examine the specific economic and noneconomic issues. It did, however, review the history of the bargaining structure and then recommended a structure that best fit the companies and unions in light of the facts uncovered and current positions of the parties involved. This type of fact-finding results in recommendations on the criteria or procedural devices to get parties around a roadblock to bargain.[11]

Finally, there is fact-finding with recommendations on issues as well as on procedure. Here the fact finders are charged with making specific recommendations on the disputed issues after establishing the facts. The procedural aspects are somewhat similar to arbitration in that formal hearings usually occur and the fact finder may believe that it is improper to confer with one party in the absence of the other. After the fact finder has secured the facts through evidence and testimony, he or she will prepare a set of recommendations that are not binding on the parties. This is, in effect, the manner in which boards of inquiry operate in the health care industry.

In most cases, the recommendations of fact-finding panels are only advisory, but they are sometimes made public by either the fact finder or the parties. When the findings of the panel are made public, it is hoped that public opinion will cause the parties to resolve the dispute.[12]

Although the fact finder's recommendations are merely that—recommendations—both parties, at least theoretically, have an obligation to attempt to arrive at an agreement based on the recommendations. In fact, it has been held that an employer has an obligation to bargain in good faith following the issuance of the fact finder's recommendation.[13]

Fact-finding with recommendations allows the parties to review their positions in relation to the recommendations set forth by the fact finder. It should be clear that either party, or both parties, could reject the recommendations.

Conventional Interest Arbitration

Conventional interest arbitration involves the establishment of a panel or a single arbitrator whose recommendations go far beyond those of mediators or fact finders—they are final and binding. This neutral person or committee reviews the facts much like a fact finder and issues a decision for settlement on all outstanding issues. In most cases, such panels or individuals make decisions in terms of adjustment, accommodation, and acceptability, rather than win-lose. The arbitrator in many cases may seek to achieve compromises between the positions of the parties.

Conventional interest arbitration has been opposed on the grounds that if either party anticipates that it will get more from an arbitrator than through negotiations, that party will avoid the necessary trade-offs and compromises inherent in good-faith collective bargaining. It has been argued that interest arbitration stifles negotiations. The system's opponents point out that both parties make a sham of bargaining because they are hesitant to make even a modest offer for fear of raising the bargaining floor from which the arbitrator begins deliberations. As Lloyd Reynolds, an early observer, pointed out, "Under free collective bargaining final authority rests with union and management officials. Their freedom includes freedom to disagree with the consequent risks of strikes. The possibility of a strike . . . hangs over every bargaining conference, and without it, bargaining would have little meaning." Compulsory arbitration, he notes, "leads . . . to a withering away of collective bargaining and the assumption of full government control of the wages and conditions of employment. . . . If collective bargaining is desirable, one must accept the occasional inconvenience caused by work stoppages."[14]

Still others oppose binding arbitration inasmuch as the arbitrator may issue a monetary award that is binding on the parties but not necessarily on the public or third-party payers.

Final-Offer Arbitration

Final-offer arbitration, also referred to as last-offer, final-position, and forced-choice arbitration, is, among other things, a process whereby an arbitrator chooses between the final offers of the two parties involved. In this process, final positions of the parties to unresolved issues are presented to the arbitrator. The arbitrator must decide between the two. The process offers no flexibility to vary items within the package or to modify terms presented by the parties to what the arbitrator might consider more fair and reasonable. Such rigid final-offer procedures usually require that the parties' final offers be certified in writing in advance of the arbitration procedure and cannot be changed later. It has been noted that such a draconian procedure may discourage a resort to arbitration and force more voluntary settlements during negotiations.[15] Many arbitrators have objected to rigid final-offer proceedings on the basis of the inflexible choice thrust upon the arbitrator to select from the parties' alternative settlement packages the one that seems to be most appropriate based on the facts and, in some instances, only on one or two important points. It is winner take all! Enormous risks are indeed involved in this procedure, but there are also possible benefits. Final-offer arbitration attempts to motivate the parties to develop more reasonable positions prior to the arbitrator's decision. In theory, the parties, in an effort to win the arbitrator's approval, should be so close together that they will either reach settlement on their own or narrow the area of disagreement to such an extent that the arbitrator's award, no matter which package is chosen, will be a reasonable one. Fear that the arbitrator will select the other party's offer causes a mechanism likened to a strike by creating the possibility of severe financial impacts due to continued disagreement.[16]

Another form of final-offer arbitration provides more flexibility. The arbitrator makes an award on each separate issue. Currently, the last-offer-by-issue system is provided for by the Policemen's and Firemen's Act of 1972 in Michigan and the Public Employment Relations Act of 1974 in Iowa. Major league baseball has also voluntarily adopted this system for the resolution of salary disputes. In Michigan, the parties may submit or change their final offers during the hearing or wait until the close of the hearing to submit a final offer. A final-offer statute in New Jersey was held by the new Jersey Supreme Court to permit changes in the parties' economic package offers during the proceedings.[17] Issue-by-issue final-offer arbitration permits flexibility and prevents a winner-take-all solution, which is destructive to the overall collective bargaining relationship.

Still another form of final-offer arbitration provides for a third choice in addition to the employer's final offer of settlement and the union's. This added choice is the recommendation of prior fact-finding panels. The arbitrator using this procedure has a strong though not invariable tendency to take the earlier fact finder's recommendations as a basis for settlement.[18]

Mediation-Arbitration

Mediation-arbitration (med-arb) offers the best of all worlds, or at least it appears to. It combines the role of the mediator with that of the arbitrator. This individual participates throughout the negotiations in anticipation of the possibility of an impasse. The mediator-arbitrator's efforts are directed toward producing a settlement; therefore, he or she acts in the traditional *role* of a mediator. Failing in that role at a specific point (and only the experienced mediator can identify this point), he or she assumes the role of an arbitrator. The obvious advantage in med-arb is that the individual, the neutral third party, who must finally assume the role of arbitrator, is fully cognizant and has broad appreciation of events preceding the impasse. The mediator-arbitrator can therefore evaluate the importance of positions and make a valid judgment as to which issues are truly critical.

This process was developed during negotiations between the California Nurses Association (CNA) and hospitals in the San Francisco Bay Area. The parties voluntarily accepted it in place of a strike. It proved a successful alternative.

These negotiations took place in 1970–1971. Interestingly, the CNA was pleased with the results, but hospital management representatives were not and refused to use the process during negotiations taking place in 1974. These negotiations ended in a three-week strike.

The third party in med-arb serves primarily as a mediator, and only after all mediation efforts fail is a final and binding decision made on all unresolved issues. Every effort is made to enable the parties to reach an agreement on their own. It is during this period that the mediator establishes neutrality and gains the respect of the parties, two achievements that are essential to the success of his or her later role as an arbitrator. Of course, the parties have a strong incentive to settle their differences on their own, for they know that if they fail to do so, the mediator-arbitrator will make an agreement for them.

The role of med-arb is a complex and demanding one, requiring far more sophistication than needed to play either role separately. There are risks, as one observer points out:

> Although mediators and arbitrators are both in the business of resolving disputes, some successful arbitrators do not possess the skills, abilities and characteristics to effectively function as mediators, and the converse is true for mediators. Med-Arbiters must be able to gain the trust and respect of the parties in a negotiating setting, especially where their presence has been mandated by an outside administrative agency. This requires an understanding of contract negotiations, a sense of timing, and the ability to induce the parties to change their positions through reasoning and persuasion. In addition, where mediation techniques prove unsuccessful, the Med-Arbiter may be required to make face-to-face, on-the-spot decisions after providing the parties with an opportunity to fully present their arguments. Mediators and arbitrators, by virtue of a need to maintain their neutrality and acceptability, are well aware of the risks attended to functioning in the emotion-laden atmosphere of contract negotiations. Because of the high visibility of contract negotiations, neutrals must consider the potential effects of their involvement in a Med-Arb proceeding on their continued acceptability to the labor and management communities.[19]

A Sober Look at Health Care Strike Options

Arvid Anderson, chairman of the Office of Collective Bargaining in New York City, wrote: "I am under no illusion that there can be an absolute guarantee against strikes in a free society, or that arbitration is a panacea for all collective bargaining problems. But I do believe that we can substitute the rule of reason for trial by combat, that we can use the power of persuasion rather than the persuasion of power to settle disputes, and that interest arbitration is by far a better way to resolve public sector bargaining impasses."[20] Anderson's eloquent statement reflects an enlightened view of the troubled collective bargaining arena in the health care industry. Interest arbitration may well be the answer.

The most preferred method for the resolution of disputes between unions and employees is the collective bargaining process. During collective bargaining negotiations, one party may threaten the other with a work stoppage or lockout for the purpose of making the price of disagreement greater than that of agreement. The use of arbitration for dispute resolution precludes the use of these economic weapons by either side. Moreover, arbitration does not preclude collective bargaining, to wit:

> Collective bargaining promotes labor peace because the affected parties have the capacity to express their concerns and the ability to have an impact upon the decision-making process on issues that vitally concern them. Arbitration does not limit this discussion, which is a prerequisite to the final step of an arbitrator's determination. The ultimate mechanism for resolving a dispute is the only procedural change. The parties retain their capacity to put forth their positions on conditions of employment. They merely lose ultimate economic control in the current round of negotiations to determine the outcome, should impasse occur. Furthermore, continued input occurs during the tripartite arbitration panel discussions, where both parties designate an arbitrator. Non-neutral arbitrators educate the arbitrator and attempt to form a consensus to reach an agreement. The give and take of collective bargaining continues even under arbitration through party representatives.[21]

The threat of strike imposes various potential costs on both parties. These potential costs act as incentives for the parties to reach settlement. The parties should then develop a range of potential settlements that they both consider preferable to strike. The range of potential settlements is called a "contract zone."[22]

> Assuming that arbitration does not impose any direct costs on the parties, it must create (define) a contract zone through a mechanism that is fundamentally different from that of a strike. The major source of arbitration leverage is derived from the uncertainty of the parties regarding the behavior of the arbitrator: the parties are willing to give up some of the expected gains from an arbitrated settlement in order to avoid the attendant uncertainty.[23]

The uncertainty of an award has been defined as "the probability that interest arbitration would result in an outcome to a party less desirable than the party could have obtained through a bilateral settlement."[24] The chilling or narcotic effect of arbitration on the collective bargaining process is related to the degree of uncertainty associated with the method of arbitration to be used. If the parties believe that the cost of disagreement is less because of the compromise nature of the method, they will be more likely to use that method, thus creating a chilling or narcotic effect on the bargaining process.

Each type of interest arbitration has varying degrees of uncertainties. The nature of mediation-arbitration requires the individual involved to act both as a mediator and as an arbitrator, if necessary. Mediation requires the direct exchange of information between the potential arbitrator and the parties. The parties may then become familiar with the reasoning process of the potential arbitrator, thus reducing the uncertainty associated with a potential arbitration award.[25] "These considerations suggest that, in order to preserve the uncertainty surrounding the arbitration process and to encourage real bargaining, allowing the arbitrator to act as a mediator and other mechanisms that provide flows of information from the arbitrator to the parties will be counterproductive."[26]

In many cases, an arbitrator attempts to mediate a settlement between the parties prior to proceeding with conventional interest arbitration. The actual arbitration process is basically the same in both methods. (See Appendix B at the end of Part One.)

The degree of uncertainty attributed to conventional interest arbitration is minimal due to its compromising nature. When asked whether conventional interest arbitration resulted in compromise, Jesse Simons, a well-known arbitrator, replied, "I believe in most instances the arbitrator or panel obtains from the employer what it can afford to give and from the union what its members want and then compromise."[27]

A 1978 laboratory simulation study of the relative impact of final-offer and conventional arbitration on a bargainer's aspiration level, bargaining behavior, and feeling of responsibility for outcomes under conditions of high and low conflict indicated that in comparison to the subjects in the conventional arbitration condition, the subjects in the final-offer condition had significantly lower aspiration levels immediately before bargaining, were closer to agreement at the conclusion of the bargaining, and felt a greater personal responsibility for the outcome of the negotiations.[28]

The overall use of conventional arbitration is greater than final-offer arbitration, thus indicating less of an incentive to reach a negotiated agreement in systems using conventional interest arbitration.

The state of Michigan provides an interesting comparison between conventional and final-offer arbitration. The state used conventional arbitration from 1969 until 1972 for impasses involving police, firefighters, and deputy sheriffs. Since 1972, final-offer arbitration has been used for economic matters. Under the conventional arbitration system, 39 percent of all arbitration petitions were settled prior to an award being issued, and under the final-offer arbitration system, 61 percent of all arbitration petitions were settled prior to an award being issued.[29]

The uncertainty associated with the last-offer-by-issue system of interest arbitration is similar to that of conventional interest arbitration. Negotiators from either side usually expect the arbitrator to issue an award favoring some of its demands and some of its opponent's demands. The award would therefore compromise the interests of both parties, making the cost of disagreeing with the opponent less than the cost of agreeing. The difference between the last offers of the parties in this system at the end of the negotiations is also expected to be large.[30]

A laboratory simulation test of the impact of various forms of arbitration on negotiating behaviors indicated a higher degree of concessions for those using the final-offer system than those using the last-offer-by-issue system. At the end of the negotiations, those using the final-offer system were closer to settlement than those using the last-offer-by-issue system.[31] "The results of this research indicate that the difference in impact on negotiations between the final-offer . . . and last-offer-by-issue systems is significant. The former system generates genuine bargaining while the latter subverts free negotiations. In other words, the last-offer-by-issue system may have the same 'narcotic' effect on negotiators as that of 'conventional' arbitration."[32]

The final-offer system is uncertain in that the arbitrator must award the final package of offers of one of the parties. The threat of this type of arbitration should therefore generate concessions from the other party if it is expected that the cost of disagreeing will be greater than the expected cost of agreeing on such terms. If one party expects its offer to be awarded, the cost of disagreement is minimal. However, if the offer by the other party is expected to be awarded, the cost of disagreement is high. Negotiators will therefore reduce the expected costs of disagreement through concessions and compromises until the expected cost of disagreements are perceived as equal. The differences between these offers should therefore be small.[33]

When Jesse Simons was asked whether final-offer arbitration provided an incentive to bargain, he said, "Yes, there is a terror that the adversary will win before the arbitrator. However, it doesn't always work because occasionally either party reaches a conclusion it has to win as a matter of principle."[34]

In developing the binding arbitration statutes in Iowa, which include fact-finding, significant reliance was placed on information presented by Robert Helsby, chairman of the New York Public Relations Employment Board (PREB) in 1973. He stated that a system where the arbitrator could select either the final position of one of the parties or the fact finder's recommendation on each impasse item would place great emphasis on fact-finding and increase the possibility of settlement at that stage rather than at arbitration. Statistical evidence in Iowa has borne out Helsby's prophesy.[35] The Iowa system has provided a balance between the need for cooperative relationships between government and its employees and the right of the public to be assured the effective and orderly function of government. It appears that there is a direct relationship of that experience on the health care industry: the third-party payers, the public, and certainly, the patients.

Any alternatives to the strike in health care collective bargaining must be flexible enough to bend to the circumstances in a particular impasse situation. Genuine collective bargaining must be encouraged; it lessens the need for the extreme impasse resolution recommendations where all else fails. Longer periods of time for the negotiations of contracts may be the answer. The law provides for a notice of ninety days before a contract expires, to be issued by the party wishing to change the conditions in the operative contract. Most negotiations start later and move at a snail's pace, with an unwritten acknowledgment that "nothing will happen until the ten-day strike notice is sent out." This is often a self-fulfilling prophecy. The parties should meet during the life of the contract to identify issues that remain unresolved from prior negotiations or that have developed during the life of the contract. Such committees would operate with the goal of improving industrial relations, being fully cognizant of the effects of crisis bargaining, educating each other as to the problems, positions, and proposed solutions that may well be part of the next round of collective bargaining. Once negotiations begin, that is, the formal negotiations ninety days before the termination of the contract, the identification of a mediator-arbitrator should be the first order of business. Initially, this individual will not be present at the negotiations. He or she will appear sixty days before the termination of the contract. This person's role will be that of a traditional mediator with one difference: both parties are fully aware that this individual, at some point in the negotiations (when an impasse is reached), will assume the role of arbitrator. The mediator must become knowledgeable about all of the issues, attempt to identify common ground, and work feverishly to prevent having to take on the role of arbitrator. If agreement still has not been reached fifteen days before the contract expires, a fact finder will be appointed. This could well be the normal appointment of a board of inquiry under present Federal Mediation and Conciliation Service regulations. The fact finder's report will be available to both parties and to the mediator within ten days, that is, five days before the contract expires. This fact-finding procedure will have a far greater effect on the negotiations and the possibility of a collectively bargained settlement than reports issued by traditional boards of inquiry. Both parties are fully aware that the fact finder's report will be an alternate to their last position as far as the arbitrator is concerned. If an impasse is reached, the mediator-arbitrator, after the fact finder's report is issued, will make a selection, on an issue-by-issue basis, from three choices: management's last position, the union's last position, and the fact finder's recommendation. This will encourage the parties to endeavor to negotiate a settlement on their own. The mediator-arbitrator will continue during this period and up until the time an award is issued to try to bring the parties together on all issues; at the very least, such efforts may result in the reduction of open issues or the narrowing of differences on issues that will be submitted to arbitration.

This may be an imperfect system, and variations are to be encouraged, but in the final analysis, there are three significant added incentives for the parties to agree on their own: the mediator who may well become an arbitrator, the fact finder, and the choice of the most realistic position on an issue-by-issue basis.

Notes

1. Bernard Karsh, *Diary of a Strike* (Champaign: University of Illinois Press, 1958).

2. Edwin F. Beal and Edward D. Wickersham, *The Practice of Collective Bargaining* (Homewood, Ill.: Irwin, 1959), p. 289.

3. Karsh, *Diary of a Strike.*

4. Neil W. Chamberlain and Jane M. Schilling, *The Impact of Strikes* (New York: HarperCollins, 1954); Norman Metzger and Dennis D. Pointer, *Labor-Management Relations in the Health Services Industry: Theory and Practice* (Washington, D.C.: Science and Health Publications, 1972).

5. D. Quinn Mills, "Collective Bargaining for a New Era," speech presented at a Labor Relations Conference, NAALMC and FMCS, Washington, D.C., Sept. 9, 1982.

6. "Labor Day" (editorial), *New York Times,* Sept. 6, 1982.

7. John E. Beamer, "Fact or Fiction Regarding Interest Arbitration: The Iowa Experience," *Selected Proceedings of the 30th Annual Conference of the Association of Labor Relations Agencies* (Fort Washington, Pa.: Labor Relations Press, 1981), p. 50.

8. Reid C. Richardson, *Collective Bargaining by Objectives* (Upper Saddle River, N.J.: Prentice Hall, 1977), p. 288.

9. William E. Simkin, *Mediation and the Dynamics of Collective Bargaining* (Washington, D.C.: Bureau of National Affairs, 1971), pp. 238–239.

10. Simkin, *Mediation,* pp. 239–240.

11. Simkin, *Mediation,* p. 240.

12. Richardson, *Collective Bargaining by Objectives,* p. 258.

13. R. Theodore Clark Jr., *Coping with Mediation Fact Finding and Forms of Arbitration* (Chicago: International Personnel Management Association, 1974), p. 248.

14. Lloyd C. Reynolds, *Labor Economics and Labor Relations* (Upper Saddle River, N.J.: Prentice Hall, 1956).

15. Charles M. Rehmus, "Varieties of Final Offer Arbitration," *Arbitration Journal,* 1982, *37*(4), 5.

16. Peter Feuille, *Final Offer Arbitration: Concepts, Developments, Techniques* (Chicago: International Personnel Management Association, 1975), p. 13.

17. Rehmus, "Varieties," n. 16.

18. Rehmus, "Varieties," p. 6.

19. Jerome H. Ross, *The Med-Arb Process in Labor Agreement Negotiations.* (Washington, D.C.: Association for Conflict Resolution/Society of Professionals in Dispute Resolution Committee on Research and Education, 1982).

20. Arvid Anderson, "Interest Arbitration in New York City," *Arbitration Journal,* 1982, *37*(4), 20.

21. Clifford Scharman, "Interest Arbitration in the Private Sector," *Arbitration Journal,* 1981, *36*(3), 20.

22. Henry S. Farber and Harry C. Katz, "Interest Arbitration, Outcomes, and the Incentive to Bargain," *Industrial and Labor Relations Review,* Oct. 1971, p. 55.

23. Farber and Katz, "Interest Arbitration," p. 56.

24. A. V. Subbarao, "The Impact of Binding Interest Arbitration on Negotiation and Process Outcome," *Journal of Conflict Resolution,* 1978, *22*(2), 84.

25. Farber and Katz, "Interest Arbitration," p. 63.

26. Farber and Katz, "Interest Arbitration," p. 63.

27. Jesse Simons, personal interview, Feb. 10, 1982.

28. William W. Notz, and Frederick A. Starke, "Final-Offer Versus Conventional Arbitration as a Means of Conflict Management," *Administrative Science Quarterly,* 1978, *23,* 189–202.

29. J. Joseph Loewenberg, Walter J. Gershenfeld, H. J. Glasbeek, B. A. Hepple, and Kenneth F. Walker, *Compulsory Arbitration* (Lexington, Mass.: Heath, 1976), p. 161.

30. Subbarao, "Impact of Binding Interest Arbitration," p. 85.

31. Subbarao, "Impact of Binding Interest Arbitration," p. 98.

32. Subbarao, "Impact of Binding Interest Arbitration," p. 98.

33. Subbarao, "Impact of Binding Interest Arbitration," p. 84.

34. Simons, personal interview, Feb. 10, 1982.

35. Beamer, "Fact or Fiction," p. 52.

Appendix A

Ashtabula General Hospital

Nurse Strike Chronology

1980

July 21	The Ashtabula Nurses Association strikes as about 160 nurses walk off the job. Ashtabula General Hospital (AGH) closes, except for the outpatient clinic.
July 31	First negotiations since the strike began end with no progress.
August 15	Nonunion hospital employees protest the lack of unemployment benefits and urge both sides to bargain in good faith in talks today. No progress is reported.
August 21	No progress is reported in bargaining sessions.
September 3	AGH reopens a thirty-bed medical unit; nurses increase pickets in response.
	A nursing supervisor is found guilty in a tomato-throwing incident that occurred August 15.
	Nurses begin a series of informational picketing at businesses and the homes of hospital trustees.
September 9	The ANA agrees to drop its demand that its professional code of ethics be made part of the contract. AGH agrees to print the code next to the contract.
September 18	Hopes for further progress in bargaining are dashed when talks end in deadlock.
October 7	No progress is reported in bargaining sessions.

October 13	AGH reopens two intensive-care-unit beds.
October 25	Area unions support the nurses at a North Park rally.
October 30	No progress is reported in bargaining sessions.
November 14	No progress is reported in bargaining sessions.
December 15	AGH reopens a sixteen-bed surgical unit.
December 17	No progress is reported in bargaining sessions.

1981

January 10	ANA supporters hike fifty-six miles in frigid weather from the hospital to Youngstown, home of the oldest contract in the Ohio Nurses Association (ONA), to raise money for the nurses' strike fund.
January 12	AGH opens ten beds in the maternity unit.
January 15	The ANA polls its members regarding the direction it wants the strike to take.
January 23	The ANA announces that one of its four major demands will be dropped in a bargaining session set for January 31.
January 24	The ANA asks that all unresolved issues pending in the six-month-old strike go to fact-finding.
January 30	AGH undergoes its major accreditation inspection by the Joint Commission on Accreditation of Healthcare Organizations (JCAHO). The ANA criticizes the quality of patient care in statements before the commission.
January 31	AGH negotiators reject the ANA proposal to go to fact-finding. The ANA proposes to go to binding arbitration.
February 4	AGH negotiators reject the ANA proposal to go to binding arbitration.
February 11	National Labor Relations Board (NLRB) investigator Bernard Levine files a complaint against AGH alleging that the hospital engaged in some unfair labor practices during the seven-month-old strike.
February 18	The Ashtabula General Hospital Association holds its annual meeting and hears reports from the hospital administrator on the status of the strike and reports

from the board of trustees and the chief of staff. The press is barred from the meeting. Four trustees are reelected to new four-year terms.

March 3	AGH announces that certified letters have been mailed to all nurses in the hospital bargaining unit, notifying them that on March 9, the hospital will start hiring permanent replacements for all nurses still on strike.
March 6	A hearing is set for March 11 in Ashtabula County Common Pleas Court on whether cars must stop for pickets at AGH or if pickets are to be regulated.
March 10	AGH hires sixteen additional nurses.
March 11	After six hours of courtroom negotiations, Common Pleas Judge Joseph Mahoney issues an order stipulating that ONA is to refrain from interfering with the movement of vehicles entering or leaving the hospital premises, but each vehicle must stop at the gate when entering or exiting. Judge Mahoney also limits the number of pickets at each hospital entrance.
March 15	AGH opens its entire maternity unit.
	A negotiation session is set for March 25. Both parties in the strike clarify that only employees' cars must stop for pickets for a reasonable amount of time. The hospital administrator reports that the hospital has hired another nurse. ONA says it knows of only six nurses who have been hired.
March 25	No progress is reported in negotiations. The hospital rejects ONA's proposals for modified membership (new nurses would have to join the union but could donate their dues to charity) and a conditional no-strike clause.
March 28	American Nurses' Association President Barbara Nichols gives the striking nurses her support and speaks twice at Kent State University's Ashtabula campus.
April 7	The Ashtabula City Board of Health vetoes AGH's license application for its maternity ward.

April 8	Ashtabula County Common Pleas Court Judge Ronald Vettel issues a court injunction to keep the AGH maternity ward open pending City Board of Health approval of its license.
April 9	City Board of Health President Gerald Severino says before a full courtroom at an emergency health board meeting that the meeting is illegal and refuses to transact any business.
	Some progress on some minor issues is made in negotiations.
April 13	The City Board of Health approves AGH's license application to operate the maternity ward.
April 24	The Ashtabula County Medical Society announces, in a resolution described as the unanimous opinion of its membership, that no individual or group should for any reason be allowed to strike or close a health care facility.
May 6	AGH makes its final offer to striking nurses in negotiations.
May 9	The ANA rejects the hospital's final offer by a 79-to-13 vote. ONA's attorney says the main reasons for the rejection were the hospital's position against a union shop and a strike settlement that would cause striking nurses to lose positions they had previously held.
May 15	AGH opens additional beds as staff increase.
May 15	No new talks are scheduled between the two sides. The striking nurses plan a car wash and bake sale.
May 18	Ashtabula City Manager Clifford McClure calls for continuous negotiations between the strikers and the hospital.
May 22	The emergency room opens temporarily during a fire at the Raser Tannery property.
May 28	The National Labor Relations Board (NLRB) files a complaint containing five allegations that AGH violated the National Labor Relations Act.
May 29	Both sides meet to talk about why the striking nurses rejected the hospital's "final offer."

July 23	A twenty-four-hour examination area is established near the emergency room. Physicians can see patients in this area rather than in their offices.
	Talks between AGH administrators and striking Ashtabula nurses are broken off indefinitely by the Federal Mediation and Conciliation Service (FMCS) "until either side has a change in its bargaining position."
August 5	The hospital reopens the emergency room.
September 10	A public hearing on the NLRB charges of unfair labor practices against AGH is set for January 18.
	At a meeting between the two bargaining units, the FMCS recommends settlement of the strike. All agree that the details of the settlement will not be released until both sides have reached final decisions.
September 16	A federal mediator sets 3:00 P.M. September 18 as the deadline for a decision on the mediation proposal. The mediator releases four points of the settlement proposal.
September 18	AGH rejects the mediator's proposal, while striking nurses accept it. Nurses hold a mass meeting at Mount Carmel Church for discussion of the hospital's rejection.
September 21	The federal mediator says that a compromise recommendation is usually the last step in the mediation process.
September 25	The FMCS ends its involvement with the strike, saying, "There's nothing more we can do."
September 27	Members of Ashtabula Interfaith Clergy offer to act as mediators. Striking nurses reject the offer, saying they want an outside group.
October 13	ONA accepts the offer of a group of Youngstown-area clergy to hold a fact-finding hearing October 29, to be headed by Monsignor Patrick Breen Malone. AGH rejects the fact-finding offer.
October 15	AGH announces it will invite Monsignor Malone to moderate negotiations between the hospital and the striking nurses.

October 23   Both negotiating teams meet without a moderator or mediator. No progress is reported in negotiations.

Monsignor Malone declines to be the moderator.

October 24   Ashtabula Interfaith Clergy declines to participate in the fact-finding hearing, reiterating its willingness to act as a mediator in negotiations.

October 29   The fact-finding hearing is held, with nurses, citizens, and a Youngstown-area panel of clergy in attendance. AGH board and administrators decline to attend.

November 15   A solidarity rally at Ashtabula's North Park is held at the finish of a fifty-six-mile walk. Unions from across the state send representatives to the rally. As many as two hundred fifty people attend.

November 18   AGH files contempt-of-court charges against ONA stemming from actions during the solidarity rally.

November 19   Striking nurses deny the contempt-of-court charges.

December 9   The Youngstown clergy panel releases its written conclusions from the fact-finding hearing and six recommendations for resolution of the strike.

December 17   AGH offers striking nurses their jobs in a bargaining session.

December 18   Striking nurses meet to discuss the hospital proposal on returning nurses to their prestrike positions.

December 29   Striking nurses hold two meetings for discussion of the latest AGH offer.

1982

January 4   Striking nurses hold two separate votes on the last AGH offer, which includes a 12 percent pay raise, a seventeen-month contract, and the return of the nurses to their prestrike positions. Nurses reject the hospital offer.

January 14   Striking nurses present their final offer to AGH.

January 18   The public hearing on the NLRB's unfair labor practice charges against AGH are canceled because a settlement offer has been signed by the hospital.

January 26	The NLRB regional director announces that ONA has filed written objections to the settlement offered to the NLRB by AGH.
January 26	It is disclosed that the County Common Pleas Court hearing on contempt-of-court charges filed by AGH against ONA in November has been postponed at the request of the hospital's attorney.
February 8	Striking nurses reconsider the December 17 AGH proposal and ratify the contract. What is referred to as the nation's longest nursing strike ends after 570 days.

Appendix B

The Use of Interest Arbitration in the Public Sector

Daniel G. Gallagher

A REVIEW of the literature on public sector collective bargaining reveals considerable research and comment on interest dispute resolution procedures. Why is there this fascination with public sector impasse resolution procedures, and especially with compulsory arbitration?

Perhaps one answer is that public sector impasse resolution mechanisms, such as fact-finding or compulsory arbitration, are rather foreign concepts in the private sector. They are a major departure from our understanding of the dynamics of conventional bargaining and may generate a need to reformulate existing theories of the bargaining process.

Second, the number of jurisdictions adopting compulsory arbitration as the terminal step for disputes has grown, thus increasing the opportunities for both intra- and interjurisdictional studies of various compulsory arbitration schemes: conventional, final offer (FOA) on an issue package basis, and mediation-arbitration (med-arb). The primary concern in these studies then often becomes identification of the most effective procedural scheme. Closely related to this concern is the considerable attention being devoted by the so-called "interventionist tinkerers" to making the arbitration process more effective in encouraging voluntary settlements.

There may be other reasons for this increasing concern with compulsory arbitration. Narrative essays on the advantages and disadvantages of compulsory arbitration may multiply as more practitioners and neutrals become

Source: Proceedings of the Spring Meeting of the Industrial Relations Research Association, April 28–30, 1982, Milwaukee, Wisconsin. Reprinted with permission from the Industrial Relations Research Association. The author acknowledges Thomas Gilroy, Richard Pegnetter, and Peter Veglahn for their helpful comments on an earlier draft of this paper.

involved in negotiations that terminate in arbitration and as the gradual increase in the number of public sector laws that allow strike action permits
comparative studies of arbitration, not only with the weaker advisory panels of dispute resolution but with the recent experience in some jurisdictions, where public employees have the right to strike.

The focus here is twofold. We begin with a brief review of the effectiveness of compulsory arbitration and then discuss a few selected concerns
regarding the use and/or availability of arbitration as a dispute resolution
procedure. The arbitration systems highlighted are those in Iowa, Michigan, Minnesota, and Wisconsin. By using these states we give a regional
focus to our discussion and take advantage of the fact that, although they
are geographically contiguous, their impasse resolution procedures, which
involve compulsory arbitration for some or all categories of public employees, are both structurally and operationally diverse.

However, when evaluating the effectiveness of compulsory arbitration,
a realistic appraisal of politically and operationally feasible alternatives is
required. The common normative assumption is that the public both wants
and needs to be protected against strikes by protective service or "essential" employees.[1] Thus, despite criticism of requiring compulsory arbitration in interest disputes involving these employees, the political reality is
that they are not likely to be granted the right to strike.

In contrast, it is reasonable to compare the results under compulsory arbitration procedures and right to strike legislation, which is currently available in some ten jurisdictions. But it is not reasonable to compare arbitration
results with those under advisory procedures, such as fact finding, since the
latter exclude the bilateral risk that is necessary to encourage the parties to
reach a voluntary settlement.

Effectiveness of Compulsory Arbitration

The literature reflects different approaches to evaluating the effectiveness
of compulsory arbitration as a dispute resolution technique. In a comprehensive study, Anderson identified the key issue when he said, "We really
don't know . . . how effective . . . compulsory arbitration [is]."[2] In fact, as
Anderson noted, the evaluations tend to focus on only a few dimensions,
primarily that bargaining incentives should be protected.[3] In other words,
considerable empirical research on the "effectiveness" of arbitration has attempted to determine if the infamous, but poorly defined, "chilling effect"
is associated with arbitration as evidenced by the frequency of arbitrated
settlements relative to voluntary agreements.

Using this conventional measure of usage rates, we may be tempted to
reach conclusions about the effectiveness of the various impasse procedures

in Iowa, Michigan, Minnesota, and Wisconsin. For example, in Iowa, where the statutory impasse procedure is mediation, fact finding, and tri-offer FOA, arbitration awards have been limited to between 4.5 and 7.1 percent of all contract negotiations over the first six years' experience.[4] Available data on the Michigan experience indicate that 10 to 15 percent of all public safety employee negotiations resulted in arbitrated awards.[5] In Wisconsin, 9 to 18 percent of public safety negotiations have been settled by the issuance of an FOA package award, while approximately 5.4 percent of nonessential employee impasses were settled by arbitration during 1978 and 1979 under the 1978 mutual-choice-of-procedures statute.[6] Between 1973 and 1980 in Minnesota, about 30 percent of all negotiations requesting mediation for essential-service employee disputes resulted in arbitrated settlements.[7]

Although these findings do indicate various jurisdictions' reliance on arbitrated settlements, it is often inappropriate to compare both intra- and interjurisdictional usage of arbitration and to suggest that one compulsory arbitration system works better than another based on the extent to which the parties rely upon voluntary compared to arbitrated settlements. Comparability among systems may be hampered by the number of statutory steps preceding arbitration, the category of employees who have access to arbitration, and, quite often, the very basic difference between state agencies in reporting impasses.

Another major limitation is the failure of most studies to account for various exogenous and endogenous variables that may affect not only the bargaining process but also the parties' inclination to arbitrate disputes. In other words, the relatively lower reliance on arbitrated settlements in Iowa compared with other Midwestern jurisdictions may reflect not only the availability of fact finding prior to issue-by-issue FOA but also the considerable difference of the bargaining environment of rural Iowa from that of urbanized areas in Michigan and Minnesota. Even if such environmental factors are controlled, the explanatory power of the models that examine the effectiveness of arbitration through usage rates is often limited and erratic.

Alternatives

A few studies have used alternative approaches to measure the effectiveness of arbitration. One, by Kochan [and colleagues], used position convergence to measure the effect of the change in New York State's terminal impasse step from fact finding to arbitration. The results showed a significantly higher probability of impasse but no substantial impact on position convergence by those parties utilizing arbitration.[8] This tended to confirm prior research, which suggested that regardless of the terminal step, position modification prior to impasse apparently is limited. But such results on position convergence should be interpreted carefully since they are based on a sample of bargaining relationships where adjudicative intervention occurred.

An alternative measure of the effectiveness of arbitration is issue reduction. The rather fragmented studies appear to suggest little difference in the number of unresolved issues presented at fact finding compared to arbitration when they are terminal steps.[9] However, most studies of the relationship between arbitration and issue reduction tend to focus on the relative effectiveness of different arbitration schemes.

Once again, due to methodological limitations and procedural differences among jurisdictions, such as steps prior to impasse, two-tier mediation efforts, and scope of issues, our conclusions about the effectiveness of different compulsory arbitration schemes are limited to comparing the procedures. Among our four Midwestern jurisdictions, the mean number of issues submitted to arbitration ranges from three in Iowa (tri-offer, issue FOA) and Wisconsin (package FOA) to seven under conventional arbitration in Minnesota and eight or more economic items under the Michigan issue-by-issue FOA.

Perhaps one of the most salient concerns in attempting to evaluate the effectiveness of arbitration is identifying its effect on wage settlements, primarily whether arbitrated wage awards tend to exceed negotiated wage settlements. But measuring the effect of arbitration on wages is not an easy task. In a Michigan study, a joint governmental agency that attempted to measure this effect had difficulty in reaching a conclusion because of problems in identifying a standard against which arbitrated wages would be judged excessive.[10] Thus, in order to estimate the effect of arbitration on wages, it is necessary to control the multitude of factors, aside from arbitration, which may influence wages. The results of multiple regression studies generally show a slight or nonsignificant relationship between arbitration and wage levels, except where comparatively lower wage-rate units were brought closer to the wage settlement in similarly situated jurisdictions. Finally, the effect of arbitrated wage levels in jurisdictions with the right-to-strike option has not been explored in depth.

Thus, it seems that we know a great deal about the extent to which the negotiating parties in different jurisdictions and under various forms of arbitration rely on arbitrated awards and, to a lesser degree, about position convergence and issue reduction. But methodological concerns often make the existing comparative evaluations suspect and provide us with only limited measures of the effectiveness of arbitration. Even well-structured and comprehensive studies may not assist in resolving the controversy over the effectiveness of arbitration as a dispute-resolution technique. As Feuille noted, the same objective data may be interpreted differently depending upon personal preferences.[11]

An excellent illustration of the difficulties in reaching policy decisions based on empirical research emerged from the study of New York State's Taylor Law by Kochan [and colleagues].[12] Despite the rather detailed empirical research, unions and managements, after interpreting the data, reached rather different conclusions about the effectiveness of compulsory arbitration and the desirability of extending the arbitration statute to cover police and firefighters.

Furthermore, different statistical analyses of a single data set may produce different results. Focusing on a "narcotic effect," Butler and Ehrenberg used substantially different statistical techniques in their reexamination of the data used in Kochan and Baderschneider's study and reached fundamentally different conclusions.[13] The issue raised by these illustrations is that interpretations of effectiveness are subject not only to the practitioner community's approval and experience but also to differences in analytical approaches used by academicians who provide much of the quantitative measures of compulsory experiences.

Concerns

Judging the effectiveness of compulsory arbitration also involves some subjective, less quantifiable issues. Much of the literature, especially on FDA, addresses the desirability of structuring impasse procedures to maximize "mutual anxiety" so that the parties will reach a voluntary rather than an adjudicated settlement. In practice, this pressure appears to differ among various arbitration schemes.

The Iowa statute requires the parties to submit final offers and prohibits the arbitrator from mediating. Since the parties expect nothing other than an award, there appears to be a limited tactical advantage for the parties to hold back on an issue proceeding to arbitration.

In contrast, the med-arb process in Wisconsin and particularly in Michigan is more flexible, but it raises the concern that the pressure of "mutual anxiety" may be seriously eroded, since an adjudicative decision is not initially expected. Although disputes in both states have been successfully resolved by second-tier mediation efforts at or prior to arbitration, the concern remains over the extent to which the parties' ability to modify final offers reduces the incentive to negotiate prior to arbitration. This ability to modify final offers seems contradictory to the underlying theory of FOA, even if justified on the basis of the sanctity of a voluntary agreement.

Judgments of the effectiveness of these various approaches depend on whether arbitration is considered a terminal adjudicative process at which a final decision is expected and rendered or a forum for the initiation of bona fide negotiations. The goal of promoting voluntary settlements, as in Michigan, must be weighed against the drawback of prolonging the bargaining process when disputes are remanded to further negotiations and final offers are resubmitted. At issue is the balance between the benefits of a voluntary settlement even if the process is prolonged with the benefits of a bargaining agreement that coincides with the parties' current employment needs and fiscal conditions rather than one that is retroactively applied.

A problem that has arisen in Iowa and Wisconsin flows from the statutes' distinction between mandatory and permissive bargaining items. Since both statutes imply that there must be mutual agreement to discuss permissive items, either party can exclude such items from arbitral review if the parties fail to reach a voluntary settlement. In addition, one party may be able to impose a cost on the other party, which may be seeking an agreement on these items by using its willingness to agree to a permissive item or to maintain contract language about a permissive subject as a means of forcing concessions on other items that are in the mandatory category.

In the short run, the strategy of withholding concessions on permissive items may give a tactical advantage to one party. However, in the long run it may impair the effectiveness of compulsory arbitration as a dispute resolution technique.

A third, but closely related, concern, as Kochan suggested, is that arbitration may be subject to a "half-life" effect.[14] One or both parties may view arbitration as a mechanism to maintain the status quo. Although critics of compulsory arbitration frequently suggest that a party may achieve through arbitration what it could not through the bargaining process, little if any effort has been directed toward determining if in fact arbitration serves as a vehicle for introducing substantial innovations or changes in the contract. If innovation and change are forthcoming only when one party has a comparative advantage, then the perceived effectiveness of compulsory arbitration may diminish, especially when the party at a disadvantage seeks an innovative solution to a particularly important problem. Should arbitration come to be perceived as a barrier to innovative resolutions of emerging employment problems, the attractiveness of strike action may increase.

An ancillary concern, also involving some subjectivity, is the economic impact of arbitration. Studies have concluded that the impact of compulsory arbitration on wages is limited or statistically nonsignificant. But these studies have not quantified the possible broader economic costs. Little is known about whether arbitrated awards substantially increase the total labor cost within the bargaining unit or if there is a significantly higher disemployment effect than under voluntary settlements.

Second, the spillover effect of an arbitrated economic award on other bargaining units needs to be considered. Again, little is known about whether an arbitrated economic award results in a similar pattern for other employee units in the employment relationship or if the economic settlements differ depending on whether the other employee units use an advisory procedure like fact finding or whether they can invoke arbitration or resort to strike action. All of these questions remain unanswered.

Choice-of-Procedure Systems

A final question is whether arbitration is more effective if it is an option in a choice-of-procedure system. Minnesota management, for example, unilaterally selected either conventional arbitration or the strike in nonessential employee negotiations during the 1973–1980 period when it had those options. Wisconsin's choice-of-procedure system for nonessential employees, in effect since 1977, provides for strike action by mutual agreement. Based on the experience in these states, it appears questionable whether the choice-of-procedure approach alleviates many of the fundamental problems associated with impasse resolution systems.

According to Ponak and Wheeler's analysis of the Wisconsin and Minnesota experience with these systems, there was no mutual agreement to pursue the strike option in Wisconsin during 1978, whereas in Minnesota managements' unilateral selection of the strike option was relatively rare in school district negotiations but was frequent in municipal and county unit negotiations.[15] Although in Minnesota a substantially higher rate of voluntary settlements followed the selection of the strike option compared to the selection of arbitration, the system had a number of fundamental drawbacks which may account for its management—it was empowered to select the impasse technique, thereby giving it a major tactical advantage in being able to choose an impasse technique that best met its needs. In fact, Minnesota managements did make use of that advantage.[16]

From the union's perspective, the perceived advantage of strike action may be suspect when it can only be exercised if management concurs. As Cullen stated, "It's not a very smart labor union that strikes when management wants you to."[17]

Conclusion

This condensed review of a broad and complex issue identifies some concerns pertaining to compulsory arbitration that warrant further study before any definitive conclusions about the effectiveness of compulsory arbitration as a dispute resolution technique can be reached. But during the course of such study we may expect that compulsory arbitration will continue to serve as a terminal impasse procedure in jurisdictions where it currently exists, particularly for negotiations involving essential service employees. For such employees, the normative assumption that the public wants and needs to be protected against strike action is both reasonable and sufficiently compelling that legislative action to exclude compulsory arbitration is unlikely. However, the increased willingness of many jurisdictions to permit strikes as a terminal step does suggest that the attraction of compulsory arbitration may be decreasing.

Given the volume of research studies and experiences, it does not appear that the questions concerning terminal impasse-resolution procedures are likely to be soon resolved. Debate and disagreement will continue as long as management and union representatives maintain fundamentally different perceptions of the relative advantages of compulsory arbitration and alternative terminal procedures. As a result, the focus in the future could shift from evaluating the effectiveness of compulsory arbitration relative to other terminal procedures toward identifying changes that might be made in the structure and implementation of steps prior to impasse in order to encourage voluntary settlements.

Notes

1. Peter Feuille, "Selected Benefits and Costs of Compulsory Arbitration," *Industrial and Labor Relations Review,* Oct. 1979, pp. 64–75.

2. John C. Anderson, "The Impact of Arbitration: A Methodological Assessment," *Industrial Relations,* 1981, *20,* 144.

3. Anderson, "Impact of Arbitration," pp. 144–145.

4. Iowa Public Employment Relations Board, "Impasse Statistics: Iowa's Collective Bargaining Law," Fall 1981 (mimeo).

5. James L. Stern and others, *Final-Offer Arbitration* (Lexington, Mass.: Heath, 1975); Ernest Benjamin, "Final-Offer Arbitration Awards in Michigan, 1973–1977," 1978 (mimeo); and Michigan Department of Labor, *Labor Register,* Vol. 3 (Apr. 1979) and Vol. 4 (Sept. 1980).

6. Craig Olson, "Final-Offer Arbitration in Wisconsin After Five Years," *Proceedings of the 31st Annual Meeting of the International Relations Research Association* (Madison, Wis., 1979), pp. 111–119; Arvid Anderson, "Interest Arbitration: Still the Better Way," *CERL Review,* Spring 1981, pp. 28–32.

7. Mario Bognanno and Fredric Champlin, A *Quantitative Description and Evaluation of Public Sector Collective Bargaining in Minnesota, 1973–1980,* report submitted to the Legislative Committee on Employee Relations (Minneapolis: University of Minnesota, 1981).

8. Thomas A. Kochan and others, *Dispute Resolution Under Fact-Finding and Arbitration* (New York: American Arbitration Association, 1979).

9. Daniel G. Gallagher and Richard Pegnetter, "Impasse Resolution Under the Iowa Multistep Procedure," *Industrial and Labor Relations Review,* Apr. 1979, pp. 327–328.

10. Government Employee Relations Report no. 820 (Washington, D.C.: Government Printing Office, 1979), pp. 20–22.

11. Peter Feuille, "Analyzing Compulsory Arbitration Experiences: The Role of Personnel Experience," *Industrial and Labor Relations Review,* Apr. 1975, pp. 432–435.

12. Thomas A. Kochan, "The Politics of Interest Arbitration," *Arbitration Journal,* 1978, *33*(3), 5–9.

13. Thomas A. Kochan and Jean Baderschneider, "Dependence on Impasse Procedures: Police and Firefighters in New York State," *Industrial and Labor Relations Review,* July 1979, pp. 431–449; Richard J. Butler and Ronald G. Ehrenberg, "Estimating the Narcotic Effect of Public Sector Impasse Procedures," *Industrial and Labor Relations Review,* Oct. 1981, pp. 3–20; Thomas A. Kochan and Jean Baderschneider, "Estimating the Narcotic Effect: Choosing Techniques That Fit the Problem," *Industrial and Labor Relations Review,* Oct. 1981, pp. 21–28.

14. Thomas A. Kochan, "Dynamics of Dispute Resolution in the Public Sector," in Benjamin Aaron, Joseph R. Grodin, and James L. Stern (eds.), *Public Sector Bargaining* (Washington, D.C.: BNA Books, 1979), pp. 150–190.

15. Allen Ponak and Hoyt N. Wheeler, "Choice of Procedures in Canada and the United States," *Industrial Relations,* 1980, *19,* 292–308.

16. Such a tactical strategy also appears in the Canadian federal service, where the union selects the impasse resolution technique. See John C. Anderson and Thomas A. Kochan, "Impasse Procedures in the Canadian Federal Service: Effects on the Bargaining Process," *Industrial and Labor Relations Review,* Apr. 1977, pp. 283–301.

17. Government Employee Relations Report no. 738 (Washington, D.C.: Government Printing Office, 1977), p. 13.

Part Two
Sample Strike Plan

Strike Plan Index

About the Strike Plan

Designed for use in times of employee strike or similar labor-management conflict, this strike plan is written generically and, as such, refers to no specific union or hospital. Instead, the terms *union* and *hospital* are used whenever reference is made to the parties in conflict. Similarly, employees are referred to only as "striking" or "nonstriking." Nonstriking employees include employees who belong to unions not party to the conflict and nonunion employees.

We sincerely hope that the need will never arise to implement the plan embodied in the pages that follow. If you should, however, find yourself at loggerheads with a union and a ten-day strike notice has been filed, this manual will provide you with the basic elements necessary to develop your own tailor-made, comprehensive, and workable strike plan. No one plan can fit all facilities, but the one presented here can serve as a guide. You should of course substitute, add, or delete plan specifics to fit your needs.

Employee Strike Contingency Plan

Key to the survival of any health care facility during a strike that affects a significant portion of its employee population is a carefully and systematically developed strike contingency plan. An employee strike contingency plan is an intelligent alternative to surrendering to your adversary, under duress and out of lack of preparedness, what you believe to be a fair and honest last position. Paramount to the strike plan's effectiveness are the key objectives on which it is based and which it must serve. Specifically, the plan must strive to achieve the following:

- Minimize the disruption of patient care

- Maximize the quality of patient care

- Minimize the negative economic effects of the strike

Essential measures to consider at the onset of plan development are these:

- Stockpiling essential supplies

- Categorizing patients into three classes: those able to be sent home, those who probably could be sent home, and those who definitely require care

- Consolidating patients into fewer units

- Assigning all functions normally performed by striking workers to supervisors, professionals, and volunteers remaining on the job

Effective organization of the employee strike contingency plan begins with the assignment of a strike plan administrator, who will in turn establish committees that will be responsible for the development of major plan subdivisions. Appropriate committee staffing is obviously essential to the plan's success; thus careful consideration must be given to who will chair and staff each committee. Selections should be made on the basis of knowledge, experience, and ability in the area of the plan for which the committee is responsible. At a minimum, the plan should address the following:

- Institutional policy
- Personnel or staffing
- Services to nonstriking employees
- Patient services
- Operational equipment, supplies, and services
- Security
- Communication

The strike plan administrator will coordinate the efforts of the various committees, monitor committee meetings, provide intercommittee communication to avoid confusion and duplication of effort, and ultimately compile the written plan.

When developing the personnel plan in hospitals where some employees are represented by unions other than the one that is on strike, plan developers must consider the threshold issue of the reaction of these other unions to the conflict. Will they pull their workers out in sympathy and support? Will the employee members of these other unions slow down their activities or engage in other conflict-related job actions at the site? The status and availability of *all employees not directly involved in the actual conflict* (and this includes employees of other unions) must be known before meaningful personnel or staff planning can take place. Important to this determination is whether the other unions' collective bargaining agreements include no-sympathy-strike provisions as part of their no-strike, no-lockout clauses. A decision will also have to be made as to whether to allow members of the striking union to cross the picket line to work and the ramifications of that decision from a security standpoint.

As discussed in Chapter Two, a no-sympathy-strike clause does not guarantee that a union will not go out in sympathy, but it is a deterrent.

As highlighted in the medical services section of this plan and in Chapter Four, essential to the effective development of the strike contingency plan is the basic premise that jobs and functions abandoned by the striking workforce can be effectively handled by nonstriking workers, temporary or agency employees, and strike volunteers. If this is not the case, there can be no personnel plan to speak of, and the institution determines how it can safely and efficiently transfer and discharge its patient population for the duration of the conflict (or until acceptable strike replacements can be installed) and in-house rebuilding thereafter. To consider patient transfer, arrangements must be made with neighboring hospitals not affected by the strike that are able to accommodate significant patient load increases and to allow temporary medical staff privileges to physicians at the struck facility to admit and care for their patients.

With specific regard to communications, the hospital should notify patients, physicians, community leaders, suppliers, government authorities (where a hospital is working under government grants or contracts), and the U.S. Postal Service. In addition, a spokesperson should be assigned to report timely and accurate information to the news media. Finally, a communication network with both striking and nonstriking workers as well as the media and surrounding community should be established to report on the status of negotiations and other strike-related information.

The labor relations function during the conflict is twofold. Primarily, labor relations negotiators will try to bring about a settlement with the union through meaningful collective bargaining, employing the assistance of a mediator. The labor relations staff will be a conduit for communications among negotiators, hospital management, and the picket line. The staff will communicate developments in negotiations to management as well as to striking employees, arranging, to the extent possible, emergency services to the institution necessary to effect critical patient care, providing management with picket line developments, and supplying mediators with required resource information.

The role of the institution's legal office during the conflict includes responsibility for all legal matters arising in connection with the work stoppage and advising management as to which legislation and legal mechanisms are available and best suited for use in effectively managing the conflict.

Strike Planning Committees

THE FOLLOWING COMMITTEES should be established, each with the mission indicated on this list. Each committee should be assigned a chair who will serve as the principal person responsible for the specific activities of the committee. The committees should consist of designated individuals from all affected areas.

Committee	Mission
Human Resource Policies	To establish policies with respect to compensation and paid leave
Financial and Procurement Policies	To establish policies regarding check distribution, check cashing, procurement, and overall Financial Department operations
Personnel Planning	To identify hospital and medical school staffing needs and available personnel, temporary services, and volunteers to meet those needs
Medical Services	To determine the level of operation, personnel requirements, and sequence or procedure for closing and reopening units (admissions, triage, service distribution, operating room subgroup, ambulatory care, emergency room operations, poststrike recovery)
Accommodations	To identify and provide sleeping accommodations for staff members

	required to stay on premises during the strike
Clinical Core Services	To determine the level of operations and services available in each of the clinical core services
Nonclinical Core Services	To determine the level of operations in each of the nonclinical core services
Supplies	To establish a plan and a procedure for providing adequate supplies during the strike
Security	To establish a plan to provide appropriate security during the strike
Labor-Employee Relations	To establish a procedure for handling of all labor-employee relations issues on a round-the-clock basis
Morale	To develop programs and events to maintain esprit de corps and lift spirits during the strike
Legal	To establish procedures for handling legal matters during the strike
Communications	To develop a plan for staff, faculty, trustees, attending physicians, community, patients, visitors, and volunteers

Human Resource Policies

I. Staffing.   All employees not in the striking union will be expected to work twelve-hour days, six days a week during the strike, especially during the first week of the strike.

II. Compensation

    A. Time Records.   To be paid, all nonstriking employees (exempt and nonexempt) will submit time records to the Payroll Department weekly. See items II.F. and II.G. for specific house staff and faculty guidelines.

    B. Pay for Additional Time Worked

        1. The following employees will be entitled to straight-time for all additional hours worked:

            a. Exempt employees (full-time and part-time) classified in pay grade 8A or below on the professional and administrative structure

            b. Exempt employees (full-time and part-time) classified in pay grade 4E or below on the supervisory and managerial structure.

        2. Nonexempt full-time employees will submit timesheets and will be paid time-and-one-half for overtime regardless of pay grade.

        3. Nonexempt part-time employees will submit timesheets and will be paid straight-time for additional hours worked beyond their scheduled hours up to the full-time equivalent hours for their position. Any hours worked beyond 37.5 will be paid at time-and-one-half for overtime regardless of pay grade.

4. Employees who have not received classification will be categorized on a case-by-case basis.

C. Compensatory Time

1. Exempt employees in pay grades 5 through 11 on the supervisory and managerial structure will be eligible for compensatory time from the start of the strike to the end of the first full weekly pay period of the strike for each 7.5 hours worked beyond forty-five hours per week.

2. At the end of the first full weekly pay period after the beginning of the strike, employees will receive $_____ for each 7.5 hours worked beyond forty-five hours per week.

D. Extraordinary Performance Bonus.   At the end of the strike, a committee will be established to award bonuses for extraordinary performance during the strike.

E. Review of Extraordinary Strike Expenses.   There will be no automatic strike expense stipends. However, a committee will be established to set forth guidelines and review requests for payment of extraordinary strike-related expenses incurred by employees during the strike. The recommendation of this committee will be sent for final approval to the appropriate senior manager or chair.

F. House Staff.   House staff will receive regular pay. They will not be required to submit timesheets.

G. Faculty

1. Faculty classified at the assistant professor level and above will not be eligible for overtime or compensatory time and thus will not be required to submit timesheets.

2. Faculty classified below the assistant professor level who work additional hours will be eligible for straight-time pay for additional time worked and thus will be required to submit timesheets reflecting hours worked, authorized by the head of the home department and the department where assigned.

H. Medical Students.   Medical students are available for assignment during the strike as needed and will be paid at the rate of $_____ per hour. Exceptions to this rate will require the signature of a senior manager and the director of human resources.

I. Temporary Assistance.   To facilitate the use and payment of agency temporaries and nonhospital employees during a strike, the Financial Division will create special department numbers so that the fees for these services can be charged.

1. Agency Temps.   The Recruitment and Staffing Office coordinates with temporary agencies and the Personnel Assignment Desk the number of agency temps, shifts, and areas of assignment. All agency temps are processed and delivered to their assigned areas by the Recruitment and Staffing staff. Agency temporaries will be given timesheets (different color sheets for each agency) and temporary IDs by the Recruitment and Staffing Office. Completed timesheets are returned to the Recruitment and Staffing Office on the Monday morning following the pay period. Fees for the agency temps are charged to the special department number created by Finance.

2. Hiring Temps.   Department heads that find it necessary to use nonstaff should hire these individuals as *temporary employees for less than three months.* These individuals will be processed under a modified hiring process, which includes a job application, 1-9 authorization, W-4 form, temporary work form, and waiver form for signature describing the hiring process. If an employee remains on the job longer than three months, a complete hiring process, including a health screening and security check, will be conducted. Individuals will be paid an hourly rate, within the range of $_____ to $_____. Exceptions to this rate will require the approval of Compensation. Pay will be processed as outlined in section II.A.

III. Sick Pay

A. Striking union employees will not be eligible for sick time pay during the strike.

B. All employees who are eligible for workers' compensation or disability during the strike period will receive payments.

IV. Vacation

A. A moratorium on vacation begins with receipt of the strike notice. From this time until the end of the strike, no vacation time should be taken. Exceptions to this provision are to be approved by a senior manager or the department chair.

B. Vacation advances processed before the strike will be reviewed and reevaluated by senior management.

C. Employees on vacation may be called back to work before or during the strike.

V. Personnel Action Freeze During Strike.   A moratorium on the processing of personnel actions, exclusive of new hires, terminations, and leaves, will be in effect for the duration of the strike.

VI. Transition Period Following Strike.   The goal of the hospital is to return to a normal operational schedule as quickly as possible after the strike. Employees may be asked to work overtime, be recalled from vacations, or be temporarily reassigned during the transition period.

Financial Policies and Procedures

I. Institutional Policies

   A. Payroll

      1. Staffing.   To ensure that all employees get paid, the Payroll Office will be staffed by Finance Personnel.

      2. Check Distribution

         a. Striking Union Employee Payroll (*location*)

            i. Check distribution by the Financial Division

            ii. Security to provide coverage during distribution

            iii. Human Resources will provide personnel to issue temporary IDs to striking employees that do not have their IDs. No paycheck will be released to striking employees at the Payroll Office (*location*).

         b. All Other Payroll

            i. All other payroll will be distributed through normal procedures.

            ii. Weekly payroll on Wednesday, 4 P.M.

            iii. Biweekly payroll on the appropriate Thursday, 4 P.M.

         c. Checks will be distributed by Payroll/Financial Division staff. Security to provide coverage during distribution. Call extension _____ for more information.

      3. Check Cashing.   Check cashing services for working employees will be provided through normal procedures. Employees will be required to show IDs to cash paychecks.

B. Reporting Time Worked During Strike

1. Weekly Employees

   a. Nonunion employees should continue to use badge readers.

   b. All others should use timecards to record hours worked.

2. Biweekly Employees

   a. Payroll will provide preprinted individual timesheets and instructions to be used by each employee working during a strike.

   b. Timesheets with instructions will be issued once strike notice is given.

C. Other Payroll

1. Salary Distribution

   a. All hours worked (regular and overtime) will be charged to the home department.

   b. Payroll timesheets may be used to reallocate actual strike hours and dollars to the departments where worked.

2. Vacation Pay

   a. All vacation pay requests submitted to the Payroll Department prior to the strike will be reviewed and reevaluated for approval by the department's vice president or chair.

   b. All requests for vacation pay after the strike has commenced will be processed only if they are approved by a vice president or the department chair and, in the case of striking union employees, reviewed by the Labor Relations Department.

3. Payroll Inquiries.   Payroll inquiries by striking union members will be accepted only by telephone. No striking union members will be allowed in the Payroll area during a strike.

D. Procurement

1. Order Processing.   Purchasing requests should be limited to emergencies only and will be reviewed on an individual basis. Requisitioners should plan their purchasing accordingly, since deliveries may be curtailed during a strike.

2. Payment Processing (including check requests)

    a. Procurement staff will process the following for payment, in order of priority:

      i. Strike-related expenses

      ii. Emergency rush checks

      iii. Utilities, leases, mortgages

      iv. Patient refunds

    b. Any other processing will be handled on an individual review basis as time and staff permit.

    c. Checks generated will be released in the usual manner, based on cash flow situations.

    d. If there are emergency situations or check requests, please contact Procurement Services.

    e. If there is a credit hold, please call the Credit Hold Beeper at _____. This beeper is for the *exclusive use* of the department to inform Procurement of *credit holds.*

E. Patient Accounts

  1. Patient Accounts will continue to screen patients financially and bill on a priority basis.

  2. Cashiering functions will continue as close to normal as possible.

F. Fund Accounting.   Requests for processing (purchase order, check requests, and so on) should be limited to emergencies only. They will be reviewed on an individual basis.

G. Other Finance Areas

  1. Third-Party Reimbursement Department.   This department will operate at a minimum level during a strike. Staff will first be reassigned to Finance functions (such as Payroll) that must continue during a strike. Any remaining staff will be released to the manpower pool.

  2. Budget Department.   Same as Third-Party Reimbursement Department.

  3. General Accounting

    a. All checks and cash received will be deposited.

    b. Swing staff will work on financial statements when not in Payroll or Accounts Payable.

4. Investment Services.   This department will operate with minimum services. Remaining staff will assist with Finance functions. Any further remaining staff will be released to the manpower pool.

II. Policies Internal to the Financial Division

A. Mail

1. Mailroom personnel will sort out Financial Division mail, and a security guard will escort Financial Division personnel in daily deliveries.

2. Outgoing mail will be hand-stamped and mailed directly by Financial Division personnel in the event that the mailroom cannot send out mail directly.

B. Bank Deposits.   Bank deposits for Patient Accounts and Finance will be made daily.

Personnel Plan

I. Personnel Needs and Availability

   A. Personnel needs are assessed at the care center or department level, following an internal evaluation of available resources. This assessment considers two different scenarios: brief interruptions (one to two days) and extended interruptions (greater than two days). Managers are encouraged to formalize employee-sharing arrangements with employees from other departments and department heads.

   B. The remaining needs are defined and submitted to the Personnel Planning Subcommittee. Information is requested regarding specific skills and hours of work for which coverage is needed (see Exhibit 1 and Exhibit 2). These are then compiled and matched with information regarding personnel, which is available to the general pool for reassignment.

   C. Whenever possible, individuals are assigned to specific departments or care centers one week in advance of the expected interruption, in order to facilitate an appropriate orientation and training process.

   D. A survey will be used to define personnel needs and available resources. Compilation of the results will be completed by *date.*

II. Volunteer Community

   A. In the event of an extended strike, it is critical to encourage our volunteer community, including trustees and current and previous volunteers, to contribute their time to help the institution maintain essential services. A letter will be available for mailing on or around *date* to solicit the volunteer services of each member

EXHIBIT 1

Sample Memo

To: Department Heads
        Administrators
From:
Date:
Re: Strike Planning

Contract negotiations are currently in progress. Although we are hopeful of a timely resolution to the discussions, it is nevertheless necessary to prepare for the possibility of a strike this coming *date or month*.

An important step in planning for a possible strike is to assess staffing resources and needs. Enclosed for your consideration and completion are two documents, a personnel needs survey and an inventory of available personnel, that will be critical to establishing a centralized personnel pool in the event of a strike.

1. Personnel Needs Survey

Most if not all departments are expected to remain operational during a work stoppage. To the extent possible, department heads should make their own arrangements for coverage by using nonunion employees from their own departments, with additional help from other departments as needed.

We encourage you to identify these nonunion employees both within and outside your department and to develop preliminary schedules for strike duty. Be sure to contact appropriate department heads for clearance if you need assistance from workers outside your own area.

For planning purposes, assume that wherever possible and necessary, hospital staff will be asked to work six days per week, twelve hours per day during a strike.

If you believe that you will still have a personnel shortage after pursuing the recommended strategy, please use the attached Personnel Needs Survey to identify additional staff that you will require from a centralized personnel pool. On the survey form, be sure to identify a departmental liaison who will work closely with strike personnel. If you will not require staffing from the centralized pool, please state this on the form and return as instructed. If you have already submitted information on personnel requirements, you do not need to complete this Personnel Needs Survey. (However, you will still need to complete the Inventory of Available Personnel.)

2. Inventory of Available Personnel

A roster of union and nonunion employees in your department is attached.

Please do the following:

• Update the printout as necessary to reflect personnel changes not correctly recorded on the list.

• Place a capital A next to the names of all nonunion employees in your department whom you wish to retain entirely (including expanded hours) in their current roles if a strike occurs. You may designate all or part of your staff in this manner.

- Place a capital C next to the names of employees who can be released, whether full time (up to seventy-two hours per week) or part time, to the central personnel pool for reassignment to areas in need. In the space provided, please note any special skills or limitations that these individuals may have.

Employees who will be assigned to other areas may be required to attend a training program lasting one to four hours during the last week of *month*. Please factor this into your staffing plans for that week.

Please return both completed documents to *name* by *date*. Based on responses received, we will develop personnel deployment and assignment lists for your department.

Please feel free to contact us with questions. For hospital-specific inquiries, call *name*.

Thank you.

Attachments: Personnel Needs Survey

Employee Roster

Identified Personnel Requirements

---

of these groups. The letter will describe the potential strike action, the nature of our anticipated personnel needs, the necessary orientation, and the procedure to follow to volunteer one's time.

B. Individuals who can make a commitment of ten or more hours of time per week will be assigned in advance to a specific department or care center. Appropriate orientation and scheduling can then be provided.

C. Individuals unable to make a regular commitment will be assigned to the general personnel pool for assignment on a day-to-day basis.

III. Additional Paid Staff.   The Medical Center will encourage the use of external paid staff during a strike period. Such recruitment will take place both centrally (Human Resources) and by individual department managers. Such temporary employees will be referred to and employed through a temporary agency, thereby simplifying the timekeeping and payroll functions.

IV. Training.   The training resources of the Department of Human Resources and Nursing will be dedicated to training internal and external replacement workers during *time period*. Nursing education has responsibility for orienting employees who will be directly supporting patient care, in conjunction with a care team. Human

EXHIBIT 2

Personnel Needs Survey

PERSONNEL NEEDS SURVEY

Department Name _____

Department Number _____

Departmental Liaison _____   Extension _____   Home Phone _____   Pager _____

Job Description	Skills Required	Specific Days Required	Start Hour	Finish Hour	Number of FTEs Needed for Sporadic Strike (1–2 days)	Number of FTEs Needed for Extended Strike (beyond 2 days)

COMMENTS AND ADDITIONAL NEEDS

_____

_____

_____

Please return this form to *name* at *location* no later than *date*. Thank you.

Resources has primary responsibility for training personnel who will be assuming primary business and support responsibilities during a strike.

V. Personnel Desk

   A. In the event of a strike, the personnel planning team will convene on a regular basis to receive staffing requests and assign available personnel to fulfill these requests. The conference room in *location* will be assigned full time to this purpose. The desk will be covered at all times and will be a point of personnel planning and coordination by Human Resources, care centers, core departments, and the Medical School.

   B. The Discharge Patients' Lounge will serve as a staging area for the reassignment of employees and volunteers based on personnel needs at any point in time. Individuals without specific assignments will be directed to this area for assignment.

VI. Medical Staff Support

   A. Department chairs and care center directors will collaborate to recruit additional personnel to support the operations of their inpatient and ambulatory clinical areas.

   B. The care center administration office will be the center for coordination of these assignments.

   C. All staff members will be asked to provide assistance, preferably in areas of direct patient care support.

   D. Every effort will be made to schedule medical staff hours that will not disrupt other schedules of patient care responsibilities.

   E. A profile of medical staff volunteer participation will be maintained for each department.

Patient Care Services

I. Charge.   To determine levels of operations and personnel required to maintain the delivery of patient care throughout the hospital. Areas of concern include patient assignment, prioritization of unit closures (if required), and poststrike operations.

II. Areas of Responsibility

   A. Vice President, Nursing.   Overall coordination of patient care services delivery. Employee: *name*

   B. Staff Assistant to Vice President, Nursing.   Coordination of the process for day-to-day patient care operation and personnel assignment. Employee: *name*

   C. Care Center Directors and Managers.   Ensuring appropriate staffing and operations in areas of responsibility.

   D. Weekend Day, Evening Shift, and Night Shift.   A minimum of four assistant administrators or clinical nurse managers and _____ operational managers.

   E. Education.   Instruction regarding functions of volunteers by staff from Nursing Education and Education and Staff Development.

   F. Personnel Command Post.   Round-the-clock coverage in the Main Nursing Office (*location*). Responsibilities:

      1. Place unassigned nonstriking staff where needed

      2. Assess personnel for assignment if units close and reopen

      3. Assign nurse "outside of nursing" to preferred units (*name* will contact to establish availability)

III. Volunteers

    A. Patient care volunteers will be provided educational sessions by staff from Nursing Education.

    B. Volunteers' activities (partial list):

        1. Pass trays, feed patients, provide water

        2. Prepare charts for admission

        3. Answer telephone calls

        4. Operate the patient call system

        5. Assist in emergencies

        6. Assist with patient transport

IV. Physicians' Activities in Patient Care Areas

    A. Vital signs

    B. Feeding patients

    C. Personal care: lift patients, turn, ambulate

    D. Dressing, change dressings

    E. Soaks: hot, wet, irrigation

    F. Irrigating catheters

    G. Intravenous therapy: administer, monitor, record

    H. Venipuncture

    I. Suction tracheostomy

    J. Manage nasogastric tube and other drainages

    K. Ventilator care

    L. Intake and output management

    M. Administering medications

    N. Transport of patients

V. Closing of Units: Inpatient Areas

    A. Goal: To consolidate patients and staff to make best use of resources.

    B. Variables

        1. OR schedule—number of surgical beds required

        2. Emergency department open

    C. Coordination of Closures

1. Recommendations to close units will be made by care center directors to the vice president for nursing.

2. Coordination of the mechanics of closure will be the responsibility of the care center directors within each care center.

3. Triage and patient placement will be done by a designated care center team, which will include a senior physician.

D. Notify the following areas when closing units:

1. Care center bed management offices, admitting, and central listing (care center directors): Notify regarding discharge or relocation of patients.

2. Pharmacy: Controlled drugs will be counted and returned to the pharmacy. Controlled drug keys will be kept by the clinical nurse manager.

3. Laundry: Cancel laundry delivery to the unit. Any unused linen will be returned to the laundry department.

4. Telecommunications: Discontinue telephone service in patient rooms.

5. Central sterile supply: Central sterile supply items should be secured.

6. General storeroom: Cancel weekly order of supplies.

7. Dietary: Notify changes in patient location so that trays can be rerouted appropriately.

8. Engineering: Notify regarding closures.

9. Patient accounts: Not affected.

10. Security: Secure and lock empty units; make rounds of closed units.

11. Care center professionals: Coordinate with volunteer service to assist in providing information and support to families and patients.

VI. Opening of Units

A. Recommendation to open units will be made by care center directors to the vice president for nursing.

B. In consultation with designated physicians, relocation of transferred patients will be kept to a minimum.

C. Notify the following areas when opening units:

1. Care center bed management offices, admitting, and central listing (care center directors): Admission and relocation of patients.

2. Pharmacy: Notify to return controlled drugs to nursing unit. Joint count between pharmacy and nursing staff will be required.

3. Laundry: Notify to deliver clean linens to the unit.

4. Telecommunications: Notify to turn on telephone services in patient rooms.

5. Central sterile supply: Notify to deliver supplies.

6. General storeroom: Notify to deliver weekly supplies.

7. Dietary: Notify regarding patient location and diet.

8. Engineering: Notify of nursing unit opening.

9. Security: Notify to inspect units and ensure security.

10. Care center professionals: Coordinate with volunteer service to assist in providing information and support to patients.

D. Operating room schedule will be planned from a daily assessment by perioperative care center directors, director of surgery, director of anesthesiology, and director of blood bank.

VII. Relocation of Patient in the Event of a Strike

A. When there is a need to relocate patients, the most important factor to remember is management of the anxiety level of patients, families, and staff. Constant communication must be established (meetings with staff; communication with patients and families).

B. Patients should be encouraged to send clothing and valuables home with their families.

C. Every care center should prepare a list of all patients on the floor with their current location and destination; this list should be available to the care center directors, clinical nurse managers, operational managers, and staff assistant to vice president for nursing.

D. The evening prior to the move, all patients should be given property bags that have been marked with patients' names in large letters. If articles have not been sent home, families should be asked to remove them during visiting hours.

E. The day or night staff will attempt to organize belongings in bags and help get patients prepared for their moves.

F. When patients are moved to another unit, meal changes must be communicated to the dietary department by the care center from which the patients originated.

G. New address plates should be made and sent to the patients' new locations.

H. If the entire floor is to be relocated, elevators must be blocked and wheelchairs and stretchers provided.

I. Patients should be moved in the following order:

   1. Ambulatory patients (first)

   2. Patients in wheelchairs

   3. Critical patients on stretchers (last)

J. The clinical nurse manager and operational manager should coordinate moves on the unit. Each patient's identification band should be checked against the list and destination noted as the patient leaves the floor; patient's charts and belongings should go with the patient.

K. Upon completion of moves:

   1. Narcotics in pyxis and narcotic box are returned to the pharmacy by the clinical nurse manager.

   2. Unit is inspected by Security.

   3. All supply closets are *locked*.

   4. Beds are stripped and cleaned.

   5. All keys are kept by the clinical nurse manager.

EXHIBIT 3

Patient Care Associates Activities: ICUs

Activity or Function	Proposed Solution	Hours of Operation	Additional Staff Required to Fill In for Strikers	Other Source of Staff
Vital Signs (BP, PTR)	Clinical nurses, per diems, agency nurses, agency assistants, private-duty nurses	24 hours	According to unit census and acuity; part of the nurses' assignments One RN per shift per unit as necessary; in OR, one agency assistant per unit as necessary	Medical students, house staff officers, attending physicians (personnel pool)
Intake and output	Clinical nurses, per diems, agency nurses, agency assistants, private-duty nurses	24 hours	Part of the nurses' assignments	Medical students, house staff officers, attending physicians (personnel pool)
Specimen collection		24 hours	Part of the nurses' assignments	Medical students, house staff officers, attending physicians (personnel pool)
Venipuncture	Clinical nurses, per diems	6 A.M. bloods 24 hours	One or two per unit for A.M. bloods From personnel pool as necessary	House staff officers, attending physicians, medical students
EKG	Clinical nurses, per diems	24 hours		House staff officers, attending physicians, medical students
Postmortem care	Clinical nurses, per diems, agency nurses, agency assistants	24 hours		House staff officers, attending physicians, medical students

Activity or Function	Proposed Solution	Hours of Operation	Additional Staff Required to Fill In for Strikers	Other Source of Staff
Activities of daily living	Clinical nurses, per diems, agency nurses, agency assistants, nonstriking staff, personnel pool	Concentration early A.M. 24 hours		Medical students, volunteers
Delivery and collection of dietary trays	Volunteers, personnel pool, hospital staff, nutritionist, center-based professions	Breakfast, lunch, dinner	One or two per unit for mealtimes, floor to floor in a care center	Medical staff, clinical nurses
Menu assistance	As above with nonselect menu and to assist pediatric staff to feed all patients Family members	Breakfast, lunch, dinner	Nutritionist; for feeding	RNs; NPs, educators, and clinicians in pediatrics
One-on-one care	Use of companions from private duty nurse's office Group patients to use staff efficiently High needs in pediatrics	24 hours	Two per care center	Personnel pool (training required)
Medical restraints	Minimal use; RNs to document and monitor; encourage use of geriatric chairs	24 hours		
Answering call bells	Use of volunteers, personnel pool	24 hours	One per unit per shift	Hospital staff, nurses, medical students
Transportation assistance	Personnel pool, volunteers, center-based professionals Special consideration for pediatric patients: every patient younger than five years old must be accompanied by a nursing staff member	Days and evenings; minimum coverage for nights	Two per unit per shift; for nights, three for the hospital	Hospital staff

Ambulation and mobilization	RNs delegate function to volunteers, medical students, and personnel pool	Days and evenings	As needed	Hospital staff and center-based professionals
Cardiac arrest team for transportation of patient and equipment	Nurses, hospital staff, house staff officers	24 hours as necessary	One per team	Medical students, house staff officers, personnel pool, physicians

Psychiatric Care Center

Admissions and discharges	RNs	24 hours	Per diems, RNs; one per shift	Voluntary staff, administrative, and otherwise within the psychiatric care center
Vital signs	RNs, medical students, physicians	24 hours		
EKG, labs	RNs, medical students, physicians	24 hours		
Personal hygiene, walking, toileting	Volunteers, administrative hospital employees, psychiatric rehabilitation, social service	Day, evening, night shifts	Per diem nurses, companions, volunteers	
Intake and output monitoring	RNs	24 hours	Per diem nurses, companions	
Passing trays, feeding patients	Nonstriking employees, volunteers, social service, RNs	Breakfast, lunch, dinner	Volunteers	
Patient observation (Q15 and one-on-one)	Psychiatric rehabilitation, social workers, medical students, companions	24 hours	Per diem nurses	

Activity or Function	Proposed Solution	Hours of Operation	Additional Staff Required to Fill In for Strikers	Other Source of Staff
Supervised visiting	Hospital employees	Noon–1 P.M. weekdays, noon–2 P.M. and 6–8 P.M. weekends	Companions, volunteers	
Transporting patients	Psychiatric clinical staff	24 hours	Per diem nurses	
Searches	RNs	daily		
Float Pool, Nights and Evenings				
Transporting of patients, equipment, and blood specimens	Personnel pool	3 P.M.–7 A.M.	One per shift	Permanently covered by operations manager
Refrigerator temperature check	Hospital personnel	Once a day	One per day	
Taking bodies to the morgue	Personnel pool, medical students	24 hours	One per shift	Permanently covered by operations manager
Maintenance of a clean, safe environment	Personnel pool	24 hours	One per shift per unit	Hospital staff; permanently covered by operations manager
Replenishment of supplies for the ICU cubicles	Material coordinators	Days	One per care center	
Respiratory therapy	Needs to be addressed for pediatric patients	24 hours		

EXHIBIT 4

Clinical Core Services Strike Plan

Department	Hours of Operation During Strike		Procedures to Follow Off-Hours	Limitations: Services or Tests Not Offered		Procedure to Follow If Service or Tests Not Offered Are Required	Staff Required to Fill In for Strikers	
	Sporadic	Extended		Sporadic	Extended		Sporadic	Extended
1. Anesthesiology *Contact Person(s):* *Location of Services:*								
2. Center for Clinical Laboratory Administration *Contact Person(s):* *Location of Services:*								
3. Andrology Lab *Contact Person(s):* *Location of Services:*								
4. Automated Core Lab *Contact Person(s):* *Location of Services:*								

Department	Hours of Operation During Strike		Procedures to Follow Off-Hours	Limitations: Services or Tests Not Offered		Procedure to Follow If Service or Tests Not Offered Are Required	Staff Required to Fill In for Strikers	
	Sporadic	Extended		Sporadic	Extended		Sporadic	Extended
5. Blood Bank *Contact Person(s):* *Location of Services:*								
6. Central Accessioning *Contact Person(s):* *Location of Services:*								
7. Chemistry Lab *Contact Person(s):* *Location of Services:*								
8. Clinical Immunology Lab *Contact Person(s):* *Location of Services:*								
9. Clinical Microscopy Lab *Contact Person(s):* *Location of Services:*								

10. Endocrinology Lab

Contact Person(s): _____

Location of Services: _____

11. Microbiology Lab

Contact Person(s): _____

Location of Services: _____

12. Outreach Lab

Contact Person(s): _____

Location of Services: _____

13. Pathology

Contact Person(s): _____

Location of Services: _____

14. Phlebotomy

Contact Person(s): _____

Location of Services: _____

15. Phlebotomy Services

Contact Person(s): _____

Location of Services: _____

Department	Hours of Operation During Strike		Procedures to Follow Off-Hours	Limitations: Services or Tests Not Offered		Procedure to Follow If Service or Tests Not Offered Are Required	Staff Required to Fill In for Strikers	
	Sporadic	Extended		Sporadic	Extended		Sporadic	Extended
16. Stat Labs								
Contact Person(s):								
Location of Services:								
17. Tumor Cytogenetics								
Contact Person(s):								
Location of Services:								
18. EKG								
Contact Person(s):								
Location of Services:								
19. Echocardiology								
Contact Person(s):								
Location of Services:								
20. Cardiac Catheterization Lab								
Contact Person(s):								
Location of Services:								

21. Nuclear Cardiology

Contact Person(s):

Location of Services:

22. Medical Records

Contact Person(s):

Location of Services:

23. Nuclear Medicine

Contact Person(s):

Location of Services:

24. Perioperative
    Service Care Center

Contact Person(s):

Location of Services:

25. Pharmacy

Contact Person(s):

Location of Services:

26. Radiology

Contact Person(s):

Location of Services:

Department	Hours of Operation During Strike		Procedures to Follow Off-Hours	Limitations: Services or Tests Not Offered		Procedure to Follow If Service or Tests Not Offered Are Required	Staff Required to Fill In for Strikers	
	Sporadic	Extended		Sporadic	Extended		Sporadic	Extended
27. Respiratory Therapy								
Contact Person(s):								
Location of Services:								
28. Social Work								
Contact Person(s):								
Location of Services:								
29. Sterile Processing								
Contact Person(s):								
Location of Services:								
30. Engineering								
Contact Person(s):								
Location of Services:								
31. Print Shop								
Contact Person(s):								
Location of Services:								

32. Traffic and Information
Contact Person(s):

33. Telephone Operations
Contact Person(s):

34. Food Service
Contact Person(s):

35. Library
Contact Person(s):

36. General Stores
Contact Person(s):

37. Receiving
Contact Person(s):

38. Off-Site Laundry
Contact Person(s):

39. Off-Site Distribution
Contact Person(s):

40. Building Services
Contact Person(s):

41. Patient Equipment Pool
Contact Person(s):

Food Services

Crisis Day Policy

1. Hospital administration will notify the senior food service manager on duty that the Crisis Day procedure is in effect.

2. Cafeteria staff will be immediately reviewed and assigned to the following ten positions:

   2 cashiers

   2 steam table attendants

   1 runner

   1 dining room attendant

   2 dish room attendants

   2 beverage attendants

   Once the ten cafeteria positions are filled, surplus staff will be deployed to hospital areas in need, as directed by hospital administration.

3. Hours of operation will be as follows:

   Breakfast: 7:00 A.M.–9:00 A.M.

   Lunch   11:00 A.M.–2:00 P.M.

   Dinner   4:30 P.M.–6:30 P.M.

4. Kitchen management and production staff will immediately review current menu status and select two or three entrees along with a vegetable and starch to be served in the cafeteria. (This may include sandwiches and salad plates; see sample menus.)

5. Signs will be posted at the entrance to the cafeteria reiterating the cafeteria Crisis Day policy.

6. Complimentary coffee will be offered around the clock, or as long as the crisis lasts.

7. Employees of the hospital with a valid ID card will be provided with a free hot meal and medium beverage. The hot meal will be available on the steam table with an appropriate vegetable and starch. A batch salad will be available at the salad bar. The cold meal will be self-service. Beverage choice will include coffee, tea, soda, and punch.

8. Employees will proceed through the cashier islands and present a valid ID card. If they do not have a valid ID card, they will then purchase their meal as required by all guests, visitors, and students.

9. Abuse of the free meal by hospital employees is not expected, but if it does occur, we will mark employees' hands using an invisible marking system visible only under black light.

10. If staff members are unable or restricted from going to the cafeteria during the meal period, their supervisor should send a messenger from the unit or department with written authorization requesting the number of meals needed and the names of the staff members they are for. The authorization and associated ID cards should be given to the cafeteria manager, who would then approve the request. At that time, the messenger would take the correct number of meals back to the unit or department. The authorization letter will be retained by the manager for tracking purposes.

Sample Menus

Menu 1

Garden Vegetable Soup

Baked Ziti

Roast Chicken

Whipped Potatoes

Buttered Broccoli

Assorted Premade Sandwiches*

Menu 2

Chicken Noodle Soup

Macaroni and Cheese

Baked Meatloaf with Gravy

Roasted Potatoes

Stewed Tomatoes

Assorted Premade Sandwiches*

---

*Turkey, Roast Beef, Ham, Bologna, Salami, Tuna Salad, Turkey Salad

Accommodations

I. Sporadic Strike (One to Two Days)

    A. Purpose.   To provide sleeping accommodations for staff members who need to stay on the premises during the strike:

        1. Contact person(s): *Name(s)*

        2. Location of Services: *Location*

    B. Accommodations

        1. Location.   Mattresses will be set up in the _____ to accommodate a large number of staff. Linens will be stocked daily by the Linen Department. Staff members are expected to make and strip their own mattresses.

        2. Offices.   Staff members are encouraged to use their offices for sleeping accommodations whenever feasible and safe to do so.

    C. Shower and Toilet Facilities.   Shower and toilet facilities are available on the _____ and in certain patient rooms that have been designated for this use by the care center management team.

II. Extended Strike (Beyond Two Days)

    A. Purpose.   To provide sleeping accommodations for staff members who need to stay on the premises during the strike:

        1. Contact person(s): *Name(s)*

        2. Location of Services: *Location*

B. Accommodations

   1. Location.   Mattresses will be set up in the _____ to accommodate a large number of staff. Linens will be stocked daily by the Linen Department. Staff members are expected to make and strip their own mattresses.

   2. Patient Rooms.   In the event that an extended strike causes patient floors to be closed, the rooms will become available for use by staff members.

   3 Offices.   Staff members are encouraged to use their offices for sleeping accommodations whenever feasible and safe to do so.

C. Shower and Toilet Facilities.   Limited shower and toilet facilities are available on the _____ and in patient rooms that have been designated for this use by the care center management team.

D. Blankets and Linens.   Staff who need changes of bedding may exchange their soiled linens in the Linen Department between the hours of 8:00 A.M. and 4:00 P.M. Staff may also access the after-hours cart located at *location*.

Engineering and Plant Operations

I. Purpose. The purpose of this strike plan is to clearly delineate areas of responsibilities, assignment of persons in various shifts, and the scope of the work involved.

II. Scope. The scope of the plan is to include, but not be limited to, all supervisory personnel of the Engineering Department. It is strongly suggested that those who are to be on duty during the strike report to work prior to the official commencement time so as to be available as the situation clarifies.

III. Responsibilities

A. Director of Engineering. This person will be responsible for the planning, direction, supervision, and coordination of all Engineering Department activities in the broad areas outlined here, regardless of funds or method of accomplishment:

1. Operation of all heating, air conditioning, and ventilation plants

2. Provision of utilities and emergency power

3. Maintenance and repair of structures and equipment

4. Nurse call system, pneumatic tube system, fire protection and prevention

5. Recovery from damage to facilities from any cause

6. Management of emergency repair forces

B. Associate Director of Engineering Operations. This person will be responsible to assist the director of engineering and act in his or her stead as necessary; will also direct customer service, elevators, personnel, and liaison with other hospital departments.

C. Associate Director, Facility Maintenance.   This person will be responsible for the maintenance and repair of buildings, structures, and utility systems; equipment and facilities of the medical center; gas and oxygen distribution systems; heating system and refrigeration; and transport of pathological waste to the collection point.

D. Associate Director, Plant.   This person will be responsible for the supervision of personnel engaged in the operation, maintenance, and repair of high- and low-pressure steam plants, central air conditioning system, central utility systems, emergency power generating systems, nurse call pneumatic tube systems, address-o-graphs, fire systems, fire-smoke damper controls, and off-site buildings.

E. Associate Director, Personnel and Financial.   This person will be responsible for payroll, personnel actions, budget, purchasing, and computer LAN.

IV. Functions

   A. Engineer Subcommand Post

      1. Post will be established in the Engineering Office, *location.*

      2. Telephone numbers will be *phone numbers.*

      3. Post will be manned twenty-four hours a day, with two twelve-hour shifts per day. Shifts start and end at six o'clock (A.M. or P.M.). First shift to commence at designated date and time.

         a. Day shift director of the subcommand post: *name.*

         b. Night shift director of the subcommand post: *name.*

      4. The director of the subcommand post will report to the hospital command post every three hours regarding the status of the Engineering Department.

      5. Upon change of shift, each director will brief the incoming director on the status of all ongoing activities.

   B. Administrative Personnel: Associate Director, Comptroller. Assigned personnel will continue all administrative functions.

      6:00 A.M. to 6:00 P.M.: *names*

   C. Engineering Operations: Associate Director.   This person will be responsible for the operation of the work control, house call, and elevator service.

1. Engineering Front Desk

   6:00 A.M. to 6:00 P.M.: *names*

   6:00 P.M. to 6:00 A.M.: *names*

2. Elevator Shop

   6:00 A.M. to 6:00 P.M.: *names*

   6:00 P.M. to 6:00 A.M.: *names*

D. Maintenance Engineering

1. Machine Shop.   The machine shop will answer all emergency calls for repairs of equipment and machinery. Routine service call repairs will be done only if time and conditions permit.

   6:00 A.M. to 6:00 P.M.: *names*

   6:00 P.M. to 6:00 A.M.: *names*

2. Plumbing Shop.   The plumbing shop will answer all emergency calls for stopped drains, broken lines, leaking pipes, and so on. Routine service calls or repairs will be done only if time and conditions permit.

   6:00 A.M. to 6:00 P.M.: *names*

   6:00 P.M. to 6:00 A.M.: *names*

3. Electrical Shop.   The electrical shop will answer all emergency calls for blown fuses, tripped circuit breakers, electrical hazards, broken outlets, and so on. Routine service calls and repairs will be done only if time and conditions permit.

   6:00 A.M. to 6:00 P.M.: *names*

   6:00 P.M. to 6:00 A.M.: *names*

4. Carpentry Shop.   The carpentry shop will answer all emergency calls for broken windows or doors, damaged medical equipment, and so on. It will install window and door preventive devices upon order of higher authorities. Routine service call repairs will be done only if time and conditions permit.

   6:00 A.M. to 6:00 P.M.: *names*

   6:00 P.M. to 6:00 A.M.: *names*

5. Paint Shop.   The paint shop will for all intents and purposes shut down until further notice. Supervisory personnel of the paint shop are being assigned to other duties within Engineering.

6. General Mechanic.   The general mechanic will be assigned to areas needing assistance as ordered by the command post director.

   6:00 A.M. to 6:00 P.M.: *names*

7. Refrigeration, CSS.   The refrigeration technicians will answer all emergency calls involving cooling and heating, ice machines, sterilizers, and so on.

   6:00 A.M. to 6:00 P.M.: *names*

   6:00 P.M. to 6:00 A.M.: *names*

8. Pathological Waste Removal.   Waste will be transported to the assigned collection point to be arranged by support services.

   6:00 A.M. to 6:00 P.M.: *names*

E. Central Facility Systems

   1. Steam Plant.   The steam plant will operate and maintain the plant in its usual efficient manner. It will ensure that all oil tanks are topped off no later than three days after receipt of the strike notice. Shift schedules and duties will be outlined. The plant will burn gas to avoid confrontations between truck drivers and striking employees.

      6:00 A.M. to 6:00 P.M.: *names*

      6:00 P.M. to 6:00 A.M.: *names*

   2. Heating, Ventilating, and Air Conditioning (HVAC).   HVAC will operate and maintain normal services.

      6:00 A.M. to 6:00 P.M.: *names*

      6:00 P.M. to 6:00 A.M.: *names*

   3. Controls and System Monitors.   Controls will operate and maintain normal services.

      a. Controls

         6:00 A.M. to 6:00 P.M.: *names*

         6:00 P.M. to 6:00 A.M.: *names*

      b. System Monitors

         6:00 A.M. to 6:00 P.M.: *names*

         6:00 P.M. to 6:00 A.M.: *names*

4. Telecom Wiring.   Telecom wiring will be closely monitored.

   6:00 A.M. to 6:00 P.M.: *names*

   6:00 P.M. to 6:00 A.M.: *names*

5. Digital Controls and Electronics Shops.   These units will answer all emergency calls pertaining to problems with the following systems: nurse call, pneumatic tubes, fire-smoke dampers, direct digital controls, and emergency power control systems.

   6:00 A.M. to 6:00 P.M.: *names*

   6:00 P.M. to 6:00 A.M.: *names*

6. Plant Assignments.   If the following personnel are available, they will be scheduled:

   6:00 A.M. to 6:00 P.M.: *names*

   6:00 P.M. to 6:00 A.M.: *names*

7. Patrols and Emergency Assignments

   6:00 A.M. to 6:00 P.M.: *names*

   6:00 P.M. to 6:00 A.M.: *names*

CONFIDENTIAL

a. Patrols will be made at various intervals so as not to establish a pattern and will be scheduled by personnel comprising each patrol.

b. Two employees will make the rounds together and will carry a multitone pager. Under no circumstances will one engineer patrol alone.

c. Patrols will check all gates to make sure that they are secure and check all engine room doors.

d. Patrols will immediately report any unauthorized persons or damage in these areas to the engineering subcommand post.

e. Patrols will ensure that the liquid oxygen tank is topped off by no later than three days after receipt of the strike notice.

f. Sleeping Accommodations.   Sleeping accommodations for all personnel desiring to sleep in will be published in an addendum to this operations order.

g. Institutional Safety

1. Director.   The director will be responsible for the supervision and coordination of Safety Office personnel with respect to their activities in laboratory, environmental, and fire safety matters.

2. Laboratory and Environmental Safety

   a. Normal operations and service to clinical and research laboratories.

   b. Response to all environmental concerns (odors, spills, and so on).

   c. Chemical safety inspector:

      6:00 A.M. to 6:00 P.M.: *names*

3. Fire Safety

   a. Assigned personnel shall respond to all fire alarms, smoke conditions, and life-safety concerns and ensure the operation of the fire protection system.

      6:00 A.M. to 6:00 P.M.: *names*

      6:00 P.M. to 6:00 A.M.: *names*

   b. Administration personnel shall continue all office functions and direct safety concerns to the appropriate officers.

Supplies Subcommittee

A LIST SHOULD BE ESTABLISHED containing departmental supply plans, customized for each specific area. In addition to these individual plans, the following hospitalwide strategy will be employed:

1. Each user area will endeavor to build inventories to an amount equivalent to two weeks of self-sufficiency.

2. This strategy is dictated by the hospital's desire to avoid confrontation by eliminating routine access to the receiving area in the event of a general strike and perimeter picketing.

3. Neither small-piece carriers (UPS, USPS, Federal Express, or Airborne Express) nor bulk carriers that are represented by Teamster drivers will violate a picket line, once in place.

4. Each user area will anticipate these minimum requirements and process in-house requisitions and outside purchase orders to the proper service department no later than *date.*

5. Supply items with short shelf lives or unanticipated emergency requirements will be addressed on a case-by-case basis, collaboratively by Security, Procurement, and Materials Management.

6. Requirements for dry ice (for the research community) will be met by parking a filled bulk container at the _____ dock at the last available opportunity.

7. Gas cylinder storage will be increased to the point of two-week self-sufficiency. Bulk deliveries to the "oxygen farm" on _____ should go on unhindered, as in the past.

8. Key areas that require a constant source of processed goods (linens) will be addressed through the purchase of disposables (OR linen packs, ICU linen, routine floor-grade instruments, underpads).

9. Bulk foodstuffs that require refrigeration will be queued on the _____ receiving dock by parking a refrigerated trailer with electrical hookup.

10. Unanticipated emergency supply needs should be coordinated by Security, Procurement, and Materials Management.

Security

IN THE EVENT of a strike, the Security Department will remain fully operational. The department's responsibilities will include

- Safeguarding the medical center's patients, staff, and visitors
- Screening admission into the medical center
- Coordination of deliveries and supplies during the strike
- Response to incidents within the medical center
- Coordination with law enforcement and other emergency service agencies

I. General

A. At the beginning of a strike, security officers, supervisors, and management personnel will be placed on two twelve-hour shifts.

B. A security post list will be drawn up.

C. Assignments will be reviewed daily to address changing conditions (delivery schedules, concentration of pickets, demonstrations, acts of vandalism or violence, and so on).

D. The parking lots will be closed unless otherwise announced. The intent is to prevent injury to staff and damage to property. All medical center buses, vans, and trucks will be parked off-campus or in the garage, and dispatch control will be maintained by the Security Department.

E. Hospital bus service will be discontinued during the strike.

F. Liaisons with the city police department will be maintained prior to and throughout the strike.

G. The police department anticipates the need for its own command post. Previously, office space in _____ had been provided for this purpose. Arrangements with hospital administration will be made by Security if the police department requests space.

H. The Security command post will be located at _____.

I. Security will operate a telephone information service command post to provide nonstriking employees with information necessary for safe transport to and from the medical center and as a means of communication for requests for assistance (*phone number*).

J. Security will provide control for the distribution of paychecks at _____ or another suitable location.

II. Entry to the Medical Center

A. Upon notification of a strike situation, only the following entrances will provide access to the medical center during the hours indicated:

   1. Building One: 24 hours

   2. Building Two: 24 hours

   3. Building Three: 24 hours

   4. Building Four: 7:00 A.M. to 6:00 P.M.

   5. Building Five: 24 hours

B. Persons entering will be screened by Security. Visitors will be issued stick-on passes that will be clearly visible to all working staff. Employee entrances should be restricted to *(location)* and *(location)*. Augmented staffing by Human Resources will be requested at each entrance to resolve questions of valid identification.

III. Coordination of Emergency Deliveries

A. Security will coordinate emergency deliveries of supplies with the vendor, police department, and receiving personnel.

B. All vendors should be asked to contact Security prior to any delivery to finalize details and timing of delivery.

C. Security coverage will be provided for oxygen tank storage areas.

D. Security will be available to assist in the delivery of blood and other emergency resources.

IV. Auxiliary Services

    A. Locksmith.   The locksmith coordinator will be available to respond to emergency locksmith requirements. A locksmith will also be available on each shift.

    B. Investigations.   Follow-up investigations on reported incidents will be handled on a priority basis as circumstances permit.

    C. Security Clerical Staff.   Staff will be used in preparing assignment sheets, administrative functions, indexing lost and found items, and maintaining logs and records.

    D. Private Security Services.   During strike situations of extended duration, contract security personnel may be used to augment hospital security staff.

V. Parking and Transportation

    A. In the interest of personnel and property safety, the medical center parking garages will close as soon as a strike is declared. Patients, employees, and visitors will be informed of the availability of neighborhood parking facilities.

    B. Daily situation updates and information on these services will be available by calling *(phone number)*. The status of the service will be assessed if the strike continues.

Labor-Employee Relations

PURPOSE: To handle all labor-employee relations matters during the course of the strike.

- The Labor Relations Department will be covered on a round-the-clock basis to handle all labor-employee matters.
- All strike-related incidents should be reported to Labor Relations at *(phone number)* or beeper *(number)*.

Morale Committee

I. Purpose and Assumptions

    A. The charge to this committee is to make recommendations to enhance morale in the institution for people who are working during the strike.

    B. Morale is the consequence of open and extensive communication, effective management, and appropriate compensation and Human Resource policies. Other activities as defined in this plan will enhance but cannot by themselves build morale.

    C. It is thought that counts: morale builders need not be elaborate or distributed universally to be effective. They do need to be genuine and respectful.

    D. In addition to the usual effects on nonstriking employees (canceled vacations, long working hours in unaccustomed areas, and so on), strikes occur during times of heightened stress (uncertainty resulting from merger, layoffs, budgets cuts, and the like). The need for attention to employee morale is increased.

    E. It is acknowledged that successful morale initiatives must have adequate resources and be viewed as important to the provision of care. The committee will take primary responsibility for staffing morale activities. However, some of the activities will require additional personnel (for example, Public Affairs and Marketing).

    F. We are all in this together. Leave your stripes at the strike line!

II. Programs

    A. Before the Strike.   Be sure all staff understand what is expected.

B. During the Strike

    1. Communication

        a. We recommend that the program deliberately build in communication redundancy so that all people receive essential information.

        b. Communication should use all modalities: intranet, informational e-mail, phone mail, newsletter.

        c. Establish the cafeteria as the central "communication station." It should include an information desk where staff can pick up written information, raise questions, and get answers. It should also include an information bulletin board.

        d. Establish a separate phone line that employees can call to hear a tape-recorded daily message with the latest strike updates and initiatives related to morale.

        e. Put up a suggestion box where people can make suggestions and voice concerns.

    2. Transportation.   See Security Policy.

    3. Food Services

        a. The Crisis Day plan, allowing for complimentary preselected meals, very limited hours, and free coffee around the clock, will be the basis for food services during the strike.

        b. The designated meal of the day, consisting of an entrée, vegetable, starch, basic salad, and beverage, will be complimentary to all employees with a valid ID. The cafeteria will be open at each meal period, 7:00 A.M.–9:00 A.M., 11:00 A.M.– 2:00 P.M., and 4:30 P.M.–6:30 P.M. All visitors and other individuals without employee IDs will pay regular prices.

        c. In the case of staff members who are restricted or unable to go to the cafeteria, the supervisor from the unit should send a messenger from the unit with written authorization for the number of meals needed, along with the staff members' IDs, to the cafeteria manager for approval. The messenger will then take the appropriate number of meals back to the unit. The letter will be retained by the cafeteria for tracking purposes.

      d. Coffee and punch will be available near the cafeteria during closed hours.

      e. If the strike is prolonged, a "theme day" will be sponsored once a week in the cafeteria, based on the food being prepared for the day and reinforced by decorations and relevant entertainment provided by employees.

4. Other Matters

      a. Movies will be shown in the auditorium for the entertainment of staff remaining overnight; refreshments such as popcorn will be made available.

      b. The president will send a letter to hospital employees' homes, thanking staff and families for their support.

      c. Opportunities will be provided for senior managers, board members, and physicians to greet staff at or near the cafeteria.

      d. Giveaways that say "Thanks" will be distributed at rounds to every unit or in the cafeteria. These need to be ordered in advance.

      e. Key senior managers will visit operating departments to acknowledge and thank staff.

      f. Periodic entertainment will be provided by employees, as indicated in item II.B.3.e.

C. After the Strike

      a. Senior management will facilitate and encourage people to take vacations after the strike and extend deadlines for using up allotted vacations.

      b. Thank you letters will be sent to the staff.

      c. A series of formal open information sessions will be held for all staff to discuss the settlement and plan and begin to heal rifts.

Communication

TIMELY, COORDINATED communication, addressing the concerns of numerous internal and external constituencies, will be essential both in advance of, during, and at the conclusion of any work stoppage.

The Department of Public Affairs and Marketing, in consultation with senior administration, will develop the content of required communications and coordinate with the departments that will be responsible for distribution to particular constituencies.

I. Communication Vehicles

    A. Designated Spokespersons. One or two individuals will be selected to speak, when appropriate, with news media, elected officials, regulatory agencies, and other outsiders.

    B. Telephone Hot Lines. Two numbers with rollover capacity will be established by Telecommunications, one to which internal constituencies will be directed and the other to which external constituencies will be directed for latest information.

    C. Letters and Memos. Correspondence will address and be distributed to specific internal and external constituencies.

II. External Constituencies

    A. News Media. All news media inquiries will be directed to Press Relations, which will provide information verbally, issue written statements, arrange contact with designated spokespersons, and take other actions as appropriate. Other than for specific purposes approved by senior administration (such as press briefings or visits to demonstrate normal hospital operations), no news media representatives, photographers, or camera crews will be permitted in the medical center.

B. General Public.   Inquires will be directed to a telephone hot line, which will carry a recording containing current information. Availability of the hot line will be referenced in communications to individual external constituencies. As noted earlier, this line, with adequate rollover capacity, will be set up by Tele-communications. Hot line "scripts" will be developed and recorded by Public Affairs.

C. Patients and Their Families.   Patients and their families will be kept apprised by letters distributed by Inpatient Administration.

D. Community Board.   The community board will be kept up-to-date via letters distributed by Community Relations.

E. Elected Officials.   Elected officials will be informed via letter or direct contacts with designated spokespersons. Distribution and coordination will be handled by Government Relations.

III. Internal Constituencies

A. All internal constituencies will be apprised of current information in written letters or memos that address their specific concerns. These communications will be developed by Public Affairs in consultation with senior administration. Distribution responsibilities are noted in item D.

B. Whenever possible, "broadcast" e-mail will be used in conjunction with written communications to disseminate information to internal constituencies. Content of e-mail messages will be developed by Public Affairs. Distribution will be handled by Information Technologies.

C. All internal constituencies will also be advised of the availability of a telephone hot line containing current information. The line will be established by Telecommunications with sufficient rollover capacity. "Scripts" will be developed and recorded by Public Affairs. This line will be separate from the hot line for the general public and will carry information pertaining to specific internal constituencies. However, since its existence will inevitably become known by external constituencies, it should not be used to convey any confidential information.

D. Distribution

1. Trustees: Distribution by Public Affairs

2. Auxiliary Board: Distribution by Public Affairs

3. Donors, Associates, Committee of 1000: Distribution by Development

4. Alumni: Distribution by Alumni Office

5. Senior Vice President, Vice Presidents, Department Chairs, and Division Chiefs: Distribution by Public Affairs

6. Faculty and Nonstriking Staff: Distribution by Public Affairs

7. House Staff: Distribution by Inpatient Administration

8. Volunteers: Distribution by Volunteer Office

9. Students: Distribution by Office of Student Affairs

10. Health System Member Institutions: Distribution by Health System

IV. Communication Timetable. Communications addressing the following specific situations will be developed and distributed:

A. Receipt of strike notice

B. Days leading up to scheduled strike

C. Day before strike

D. Reaching of settlement

Index

N

National Union of Hospital and Health Care Employees, District 1199 Constitution, 34–35, 45–46
National Union Strike and Defense Fund (District 1199), 35
National War Labor Board, 49
Negotiations: "contract zone" during, 68; notice requirements for contract renewal, 5*fig*; notice requirements for initial contract, 4*fig*; role of labor relations staff during, 94. *See also* Arbitration; Collective bargaining; Labor disputes
New York State Nurses Association strike (1998), 46
News Union of Baltimore v. *NLRB*, 21
"Nightingalism" phenomenon, 47
Nixon, R. M., 3
NLRA (National Labor Relations Act): Ally Doctrine developed from, 11; amendments (1974) to, 12–13; on contract notice, 4; on health care coverage by, 3–4; health care labor relations governed by, 3; illegal strikes under, 32–33; on mediation, 4–9; nursing strikes and Public Law 93-360 amendment of, 51–52; prohibiting recognition strikes, 23–24; on right of employee to resign from union, 41; serving section 8(g) notice guidelines by, 13–14; on strike notice, 9–11; unfair labor practice strikes protection by, 20–21
NLRB, Booster Lodge No. 405 v., 41
NLRB, Gary Hobart Water Corporation v., 21
NLRB Granite State Joint Board, Textile Workers Union of America, Local 1029, AFL-CIO case, 41
NLRB, Metropolitan Edison Company v., 38
NLRB, Montana-Dakota Utilities v., 21
NLRB, Montegiore Hospital and Medical Center v., 10–11
NLRB, News Union of Baltimore v., 21
NLRB, Pattern Makers v., 41
NLRB v. Rockaway News Supply Company, 21
No-strike clauses: examples of, 25–26; prohibiting sympathy strikes, 22–23; strikes in violation of, 24, 26–27
Norris-La Guardia Act (1932), 26–27
Notice Requirements for Health Care Institutions: Contract Renewal Negotiations, 5*fig*
Notice Requirements for Health Care Institutions: Initial Contract Negotiations, 4*fig*
Nurses: CNA improvement of economic conditions of, 48–49; collective bargaining issues and, 52–54; compared to nonmedical employees, 45–47; conflicts in perceptions of, 47–48; "Nightingalism" phenomenon and, 47; process of collective bargaining with, 54. *See also* ANA (American Nurses Association); Employees
Nursing strike alternatives: conventional interest arbitration as, 64–65, 68–70; fact-finding as, 62–64, 71–72; (FOA) final-offer arbitration as, 65–66, 69, 83, 84; mediation-arbitration (med-arb) as, 4–9, 66–67, 68–69; as new undertaking, 62
Nursing strikes: after ANA's rescinded no-strike pledge (1969), 51; alternatives to, 62–67; ANA no-strike policy (1968) prohibiting, 48, 49, 50; anatomy

of three different, 55–56; complex impact of, 56, 60–61; defensibility of, 61–62; distinguished from nonmedical employee strikes, 45–47; patient fear as factor in, 46–47; Public Law 93-360 impact on, 51–52; sober look at options of, 67–72. *See also* Strikes
NYSNA (New York State Nurses Association), Council of Nurse Practitioners of the Mount Sinai Hospital, 35

O

Office of Collective Bargaining (New York City), 67
Owley, C., 54

P

Patient care services: clinical core services strike plan, 119*e*–125*e*; ICUs strike plan for, 115*e*–118*e*; outline of, 110–114
Pattern Makers v. *NLRB*, 41
Payne & Keller, Inc. case, 39
PERB (New York Public Relations Employment Board), 70
Personnel Needs Survey, 108*e*
Personnel strike plan, 105–109
P.L. 93-360. *See* NLRA (National Labor Relations Act)
Policemen's and Firemen's Act of 1972 (Michigan), 65
Ponak, A., 87
President Kennedy's Advisory Committee on Labor-Management Policy, 63
Price Brothers Company case, 38
Professional Practice Committee, 51
Public Employment Relations Act of 1974 (Iowa), 65
Public relations strike strategy, 37

R

RCIU (Retail Clerks International Union), 35
Recognition strikes, 23–24
Retail Clerks Local 770, Boys Markets, Inc. v., 27
Reynolds, L., 64–65
Rockaway News Supply Company, NLRB, 21

S

Section 8(g) notice, 13–14
Security strike plan, 138–140
SEIU (Service Employees International Union), 35, 36
Service Employees International Union, 34
Shutt, B. G., 48, 50–51
Simkin, W. E., 29
Simons, J., 70
"Stock effect," 60
Strike funds, 35–36
Strike notice, 9–11
Strike plan: accommodations as part of, 128–129; on communication during strike, 94, 145–147; described, 91–92; employee contingency, 92–94; on engineering and plant operations, 130–135; financial policies and procedures as part of, 101–104; food services as part of, 126–127; human resource policies as part of, 97–100; index of, 91; labor-employee relations